Presentations in Primary Care

An Illustrated Introduction to Patient Management in
General Practice

J.D.E. Knox

Professor of General Practice,
University of Dundee

Butterworths
London   Boston   Durban   Singapore   Sydney   Toronto   Wellington

First published, 1985

© **Text: Butterworths & Co. (Publishers) Ltd 1985**

Illustrations: The various Update contributors listed

British Library Cataloguing in Publication Data

Knox, J. D. E.
   Presentations in primary care: an illustrated
   introduction to patient management in general practice
   1. Physician and patient
   I. Title
   610.69′6   R727.3

   ISBN 0-407-00354-1

Library of Congress Cataloging in Publication Data

Knox, James D. E.
   Presentations in primary care.

   Bibliography: p.
   Includes index.
   1. Family medicine. I. Title. [DNLM: 1. Family
   Practice. 2. Primary Health Care. WB 110 K74p]
   R729.5.G4K56   1985   610   85-5727

   ISBN 0-407-00354-1

Photoset by Butterworths Litho Preparation Department
Printed and bound by Robert Hartnoll Ltd, Bodmin, Cornwall

Preface

Britain is justly proud of her tradition of medical care and in particular her heritage of general practice. Both helped to shape the National Health Service and, to some extent, they have been preserved in the ground rules by which the Service operates. In this way, for example, the right of each patient to choose his or her general practitioner has been maintained. The NHS was not primarily responsible for the separation of general practice from specialist hospital practice – that had already taken place before 1948 – but it added the weight of bureaucracy to the separation, thereby making real professional *rapprochement* more difficult.

One result has been to strengthen the identity of British general practice and, with it, the definition of roles and functions of a unified primary care system: this has consequences for hospital care, in terms of efficiency, effectiveness and education. Because primary care is relatively much cheaper than hospital care, a medical care system heavily dependent on strong primary care is all the more efficient in an economy of retrenchment. By ensuring that the only problems which reach specialist care are those which require that particular resource, good primary care makes for more effective use of scarce specialist skills. On the other hand, because of its sifting function and the very great extent to which that function operates, the problems with which NHS hospitals in general, and teaching hospitals in particular have to deal, are not in the least 'representative' of the common and changing health problems outside their walls. Undergraduate medical education is still firmly and almost exclusively based on teaching hospitals, so it is little wonder that medical students emerge ill equipped to cope with health problems which the medical care system has selectively excluded from their experience (Maddison, 1978; Metcalfe, 1979; Wood and Badley, 1981).

University departments of general practice are striving, with help from many quarters, to right what they perceive to be an imbalance. My personal experience of the scene over the past 15 years leads me to take a cautious view of what has been achieved. This, perhaps limited, view is further supported by the 'conversion course' nature of postgraduate vocational training for general practice which does not naturally follow on from undergraduate education (P. Stott, 1983). This book has been put together as a contribution to promote a greater orientation towards medicine in the community at levels appropriate for new entrants to general practice and senior undergraduates.

Much has already been produced from general practice, stressing the psychosocial elements so necessary for effective management of all clinical situations and vital to those in general practice. Such approaches have contributed much to conceptual thinking in the emerging discipline of general practice. At the same time, however, if the focus is solely on those aspects of medicine – often missing from hospital-based teaching – an equally unbalanced picture might emerge. Publications aimed at introducing the trainee to the clinical medicine of general practice are beginning to appear (Fry, 1982; Hall, 1983; Reed, 1984). Such accounts adopt a traditional approach of describing clinical features of a disease under a diagnostic heading. Convenient though this is, its usefulness to the trainee in practice is limited, because the first-contact nature of primary care requires the doctor to work from clinical presentations to diagnosis, and not the other way round.

The situation may be regarded as a triangle with the doctor (D), the patient (P) and the health problem of disease (HP) as the apices. Clinical teaching has hitherto tended to focus on disease largely in relation to the doctor. The approach adopted in this book focuses on the patient and his relationship to the doctor.

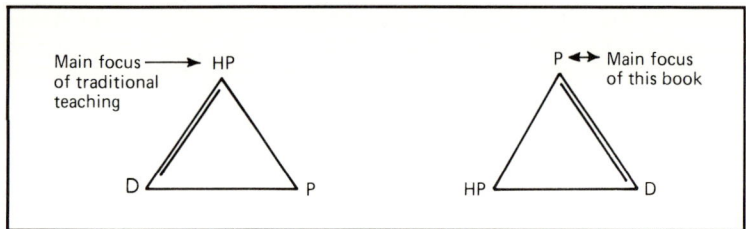

This pragmatic approach is based on a belief that it is possible to teach from the particular to embrace wider underlying principles – and I have assumed that the reader already has a certain degree of clinical sophistication. This is why many of the presentations start, not with physical diagnosis (in some instances I hope the photographs make this abundantly clear), but at a point beyond, raising issues relevant to patients and doctors *as people*.

I am indebted to the constant encouragement I have received from the staff of Butterworths and from Anne Patterson in the hard work of preparing the studies. The general practitioner tutors of the Department of General Practice have contributed ideas and comments, though I must accept full responsibility for errors of omission and commission.

The late Dr Arthur Reid contributed to Part III.
Photographs are reproduced by kind permission of:

Bevan, P.G.	Scully, C. and Williams, G.
Clarke, I.M.C.	Semmens, J.M.
Fraser, F.W.	Smith, H.
Fry, L.	Sneddon, I.
Professor Miles Irving	Thompson, M.K.
Khan, A.R.	Vanhegan, J. and Wynn-Jones, C.
Professor G. Murdoch	Welsby, P.D.
Orr, C.M.E. and Photiou, S.	Woodward, J.
Scholefield, R.D.	Eli Lilly Co.
Scully, C.	Calmic Medical Division

Miss Alison Scott patiently retyped several drafts.

J.D.E. Knox
Dundee, 1985

To
E.V.K.

Introduction

What this book aims to do

This book is intended to:

1. Stimulate the reader to think about issues not usually considered in conventional clinical text-books. Such issues include the doctors' and patients' emotional reactions to the problems presented, and the practical implications that diagnosis and treatment may have for them.
2. Increase the range of knowledge that trainees and medical students have about general practice as an academic discipline.
3. Provide tutors and trainers with a means to assess the needs of the learner.

By illustrating a few specific learning objectives in a practical way, the book may assist trainers to consider more fully the many teaching issues inherent in any contact with patients in general practice.

How to use this book

Each of the above aims calls for a slightly different use of the book, which is set out in three parts.

Part I

Part I contains the presentations; though each has been carefully selected to raise specific issues, in putting the scenarios together no attempt has been made to group them by identifiable category. Such an approach attempts to preserve the disorganized nature of patient–doctor contacts and the 'opportunistic' flavour of one-to-one teaching so characteristic of general practice.

The student wishing to obtain the most out of Part I should sit down and commit himself in writing to answer the problems set. Then, and only then, should he turn to Part II.

Part II

This part of the book is an attempt to set out some of the issues raised by the presentations in Part I. In some instances answers have been given. Some may be judged idiosyncratic; others will, in the light of progress, be shown to be wrong. Each presentation includes a reference for further study (the bibliography is brought together in the concluding section of the book).

A reading of Part II may contribute to aim (2) above, i.e. 'to increase the range of knowledge'.

Using the book as an assessment instrument

The tutor might wish to select from the index a number of issues – say, patient help-seeking behaviour, or general practitioner professional activities (such as referral), or minor clinical medicine. The scenarios in which these issues are salient are then selected. The trainee or student is asked to respond to the relevant questions, and the trainer may compare the trainee's responses with his own – and both with those set out in Part II. No attempt has been made to suggest marks for responses, though theoretically this is feasible.

In this way, the book might be used at the start of a period of training in a teaching practice to identify gaps in knowledge. By the same token, a similar use at the end of the training period might help to demonstrate to teacher and student how far specific goals of training thus identified have been achieved.

Extending the trainer's teaching objectives

The issues selected for each presentation in this book are, of course, not the only ones a teacher may wish to choose. Their choice has been influenced to some extent by an attempt to cover as wide a field as possible within the broad aims of teaching in general practice, while avoiding repetition. Trainers may therefore wish to consider for each presentation what additional teaching issues, if any, they can identify.

Part III

Part III contains short descriptions of what may be entailed in teaching and learning in the setting of a teaching practice. The issues raised in this book are interpreted aginst a background of some of the shortcomings of current medical education, and are based on the everyday work of the general practitioner.

The work of the general practitioner

The general practitioner is a licensed medical graduate who gives personal, primary and continuing care to individuals, families and a practice population, irrespective of age, sex and illness. It is the synthesis of these functions which is unique. He (she) will attend his patients in his consulting room and in their homes and, sometimes, in a clinic or a hospital. His aim is to make early diagnoses. He will include and integrate physical, psychological and social factors in his considerations about health and illness. This will be expressed in the care of his patients. He will make an initial decision about every problem which is presented to him as a doctor. He will undertake the continuing management of his patients with chronic, recurrent or terminal illnesses. Prolonged contact means that he can use repeated opportunities to gather information at a pace appropriate to each patient and build up a relationship of trust which he can use professionally. He will practise in co-operation with other colleagues, medical and non-medical. He will know how and when to intervene, through treatment, prevention and education, to promote the health of his patients and their families. He will recognize that he also has a professional responsibility to the community (the Leeuwenhorst definition (European Conference on the Teaching of General Practice, 1977)).

Contents

Presents

Part I

Presentations in general practice

Section 1

In consultation

Presentation 1: Minnie W

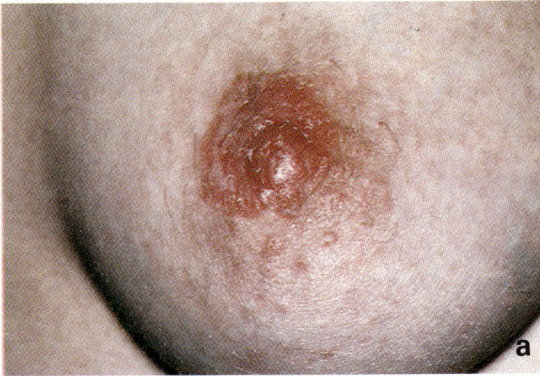

Miss Minnie W, aged 71 years, lives alone: she appears to cope well with life. The last entry in her general practice medical record, dated 18 months ago, reads: 'Small patch eczema L wrist. R ung hydrocortisone 1%'.

She now consults you about a cold she's had for a week, and you confirm that she has a mild pharyngitis. While you are making sure that her chest is clinically clear, she says, 'By the way, Doctor, could you do anything for this irritation – it's that dermatitis again, isn't it?'. She shows you her left nipple (*see illustration*). There is a sticky serous discharge staining the cotton wool with which she has padded her bra. 'So embarrassing', she says.

(a) Identify possible constraints and barriers to free communication between you and Minnie at this consultation.
(b) Her niece, Mrs McDonald, who has accompanied her and has remained in the waiting room, comes forward as you escort Minnie from the consulting room, ready to take her home. What are the pros and cons of discussing Minnie's situation with Mrs McDonald?

4

Presentation 2: Graham

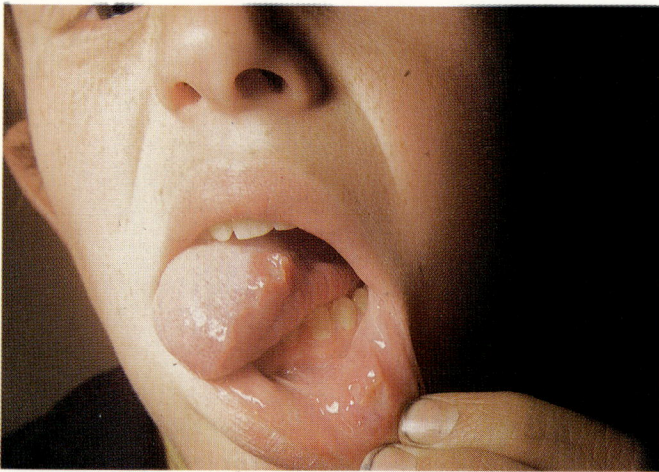

Graham, now aged 19 years, has been unemployed since leaving
school 3 years ago. At the age of 16 years he had an attack of acute
encephalitis and during the ensuing 6 months suffered two
syncopal episodes. One of these, witnessed by his mother, was
seen to have the characteristics of grand mal. His ECG showed a
'doubtful temporal lobe abnormality'. For the past 2½ years he
has remained free of fits, taking regular carbamazepine and
sodium valproate. Responsibility for his continuing care has been
passed back to you from the neurology clinic.

His visit to you is occasioned by a recurrence of his sore mouth
(*see illustration*). He also uses this occasion to raise again the
question of sitting his driving test. This is now urgent, because he
says he has been offered a job provided he can learn to drive. He
also requests a further supply of his medication.

(a) Is the lesion illustrated related to his condition and/or his
    anticonvulsive therapy?
(b) What line would you take about his fitness to drive?
(c) What view do you take of continuing his drug therapy in the
    immediate future?

Presentation 3: Jim T

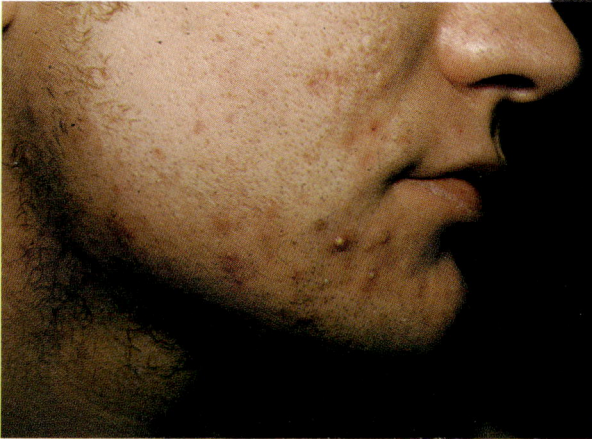

You are half-way through a morning surgery: Jim T, a computer engineer in his twenties, is your next patient. He says his spots are no better. You have three colleagues in the practice, and a trainee. You note that over the past year Jim T has consulted all the other doctors in the practice and the previous trainee. You note that sulphur and salicylic acid BPC, Minocin (oxytetracycline) and Quinoderm (potassium hydroxyquinoline and benzoyl peroxide) have been prescribed.

(a) Outline your management of Jim's problem.
(b) Comment on Jim's free movement from doctor to doctor in the practice.
(c) If Jim had *not* been consulting about his spots (e.g. had he attended for a sickness certificate following meniscectomy), would you have mentioned his spots? Give reasons for your answer.

Presentation 4: Tommy Adamson

One Sunday morning when you are on call, Mrs Adamson telephones, apologizing for 'bothering' you on a Sunday. 'Tommy, my 7-year-old son, stood on a nail last week', she says. 'He's got a sore foot and he's developed a bit of a limp.' You remember the Adamsons as a cheerful well-integrated family living at the far side of the practice area, some 5 miles away. Mrs Adamson used to work as a State-enrolled Nurse in the local geriatric hospital. You accept Mrs Adamson's offer to bring Tommy over to the surgery premises where, half an hour later, you meet him, accompanied by his father and mother. Tommy's foot is shown in the photograph.

(a) Possible referral

Using the information available, incomplete though it may be, you can begin to make some management decisions. For example, you might already be considering the most appropriate setting – home or hospital – for Tommy's treatment. Were you to arrange in-patient care, which discipline, in which kind of hospital, would you involve?

(b) Further information

Irrespective of your answer to (a), you would wish to elicit further items of relevant information. List any two you consider particularly important.

(c) General practice management

Should you decide to treat Tommy at home:
(i) How would you ensure that, on a Sunday morning, he would receive appropriate drug therapy?
(ii) What follow-up arrangements would you make?

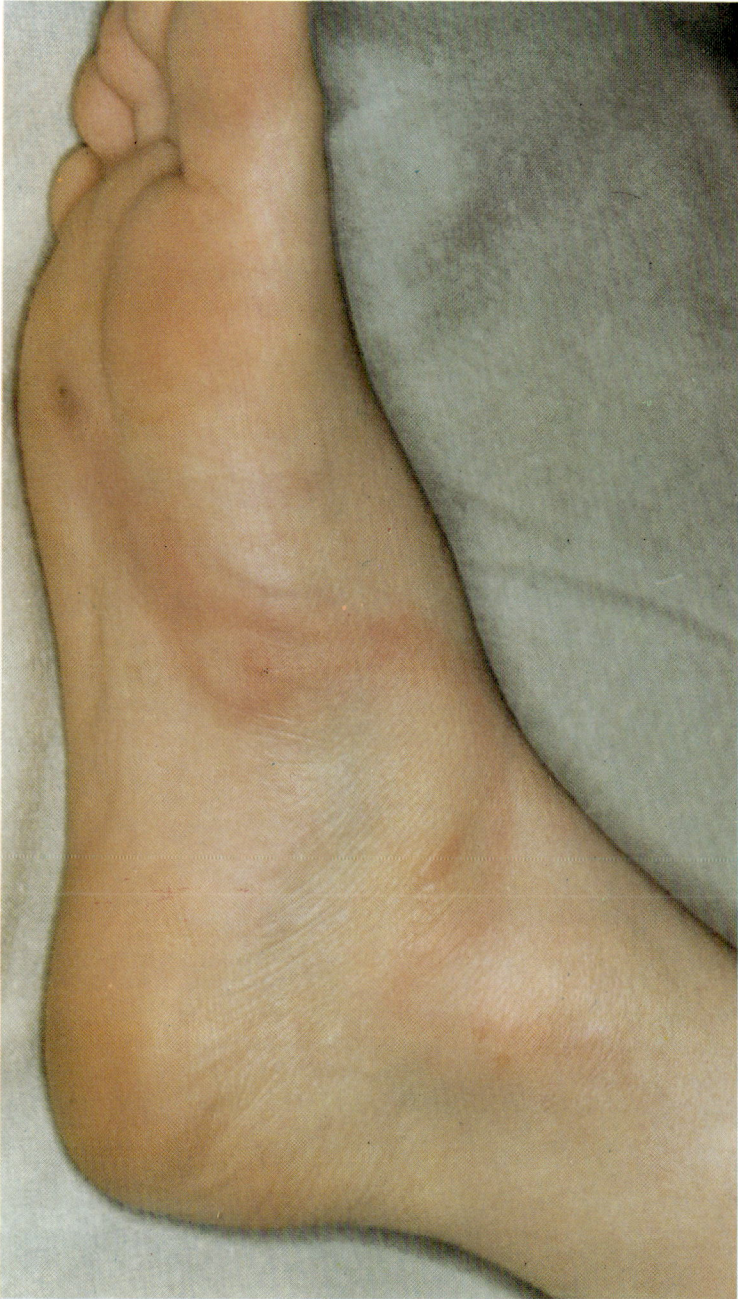

Presentation 5: Jimmy

Jimmy (aged 14 years) is the eldest of three children, the youngest of whom, now aged 7, is a spastic. His father brings Jimmy to your surgery, saying that his face has been swollen and a bit painful since yesterday. Jimmy is otherwise well and the appearances are as in the photograph.

(a) Differential diagnosis

Your differential diagnosis might include submandibular mumps. What else might it include?

(b) Drug treatment

(i) If you decide that Jimmy has mumps, what drugs, if any, might you consider prescribing – and why?

(ii) Under the National Health Service, is Jimmy entitled to obtain his drugs free of charge?

(c) The family

If, in your reply to your statement that you think Jimmy is suffering from mumps, Jimmy's father were to say, 'I'd like to prevent this spreading to Marie' (the 7-year-old spastic), what would you say – and do?

(d) Society

(i) Is mumps a notifiable disease? If so, what 'authority' is notified?

(ii) Would you exclude Jimmy from school – if so, for how long?

Presentation 6: Harry Smith

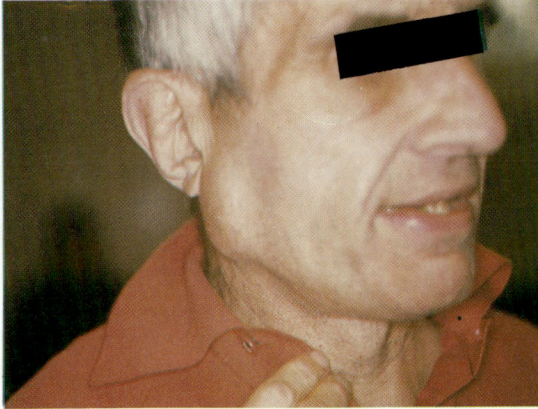

Harry Smith, a solicitor's clerk, aged 65 years, has been a patient with the practice for the past 15 years, during which time his medical record contains only one entry: 'Flu, certificate given', dated 10 years previously. He consults you, somewhat apologetically, saying his wife had nagged him to come and see about the painless swelling which has slowly developed over the last couple of years. He says he feels fine otherwise.

Palpation reveals a firm, non-tender, rather irregular mass in the right preauricular region.

(a) What does the general practice medical record tell you about Harry's illness behaviour, and how might this influence what you might say or do at this consultation?
(b) If you decide to mobilize specialist resources, which ones might you choose?
(c) What would you say to Harry at this consultation?

Presentation 7: Robert

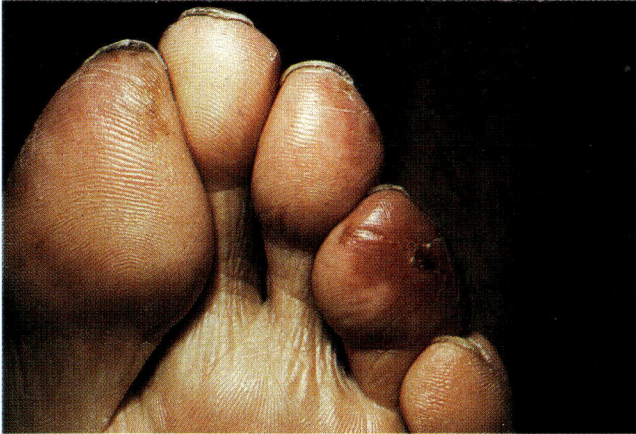

Robert is an AA patrolman in his forties. All last winter he was plagued by chilblains and now, in late November, he consults again with itchy, painful blotches on his toes. The skin of the fourth left toe is broken and the lesion is very tender.

(a) What are chilblains?
(b) Bearing in mind possible alternative diagnoses in Robert's case, what aspects of history, physical examination and further investigation might be of particular relevance?
(c) If, in the face of negative results from your further consideration, you regard chilblains to be the continuing underlying diagnosis, what advice would you give Robert?
(d) What part do drugs play in the management of chilblains?

Presentation 8: Joanna B

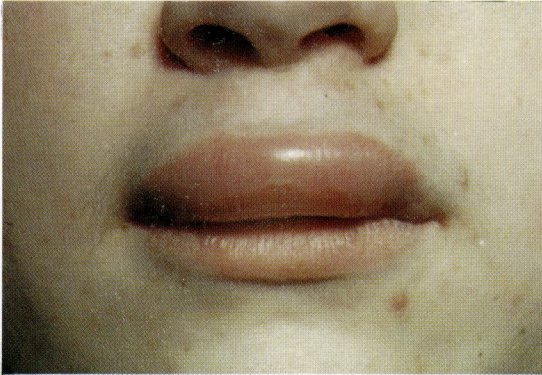

Mrs Joanna B, aged 21 years, has suffered from intermittent 'allergies' for the last 5 years. You have witnessed two episodes of giant urticaria which she has exhibited and she is a martyr to hay fever. She has been on an antihistamine, clemastine (Tavegil), on a once-daily dose for the last 18 months during which she has remained free from urticaria – though her hay fever required energetic local therapy last summer. She consults you with a swelling of her lip. And she says, coyly, 'I haven't had my 'usuals' for the last two months – I wonder if I'm pregnant?'.

(a) What steps might you take at this consultation?
(b) If Joanna is pregnant, does this influence her drug therapy, and if so, in what ways?
(c) Under NHS regulations, some sufferers from certain diseases are exempt from prescription charges. How might Joanna stand in this regard?

Presentation 9: Terence Wilton

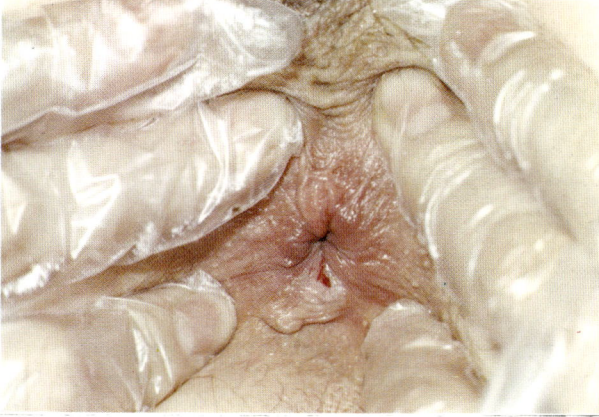

Mr Terence Wilton, a 45-year-old oil executive, consults saying 'Thanks, I'd rather stand. It's those damn piles again.' (You remember he had a haemorrhoidectomy 3 years ago.) 'They've been bleeding and it's sore as hell when I go to the toilet. I'm off to Gambia tomorrow – it couldn't have come at a worse time. You'd better give me something to prevent travellers' diarrhoea.' Examination reveals the state of affairs in the photograph.

(a) What might you do to ensure Mr Wilton's smooth passage?
(b) The doctor is wearing plastic gloves: how are these obtained, and disposed of, in general practice?
(c) How might Mr Wilton obtain advice about inoculation and health requirements for travelling abroad? Is he entitled to 'something for travellers' diarrhoea' under NHS regulations?

Presentation 10: Mr Gray

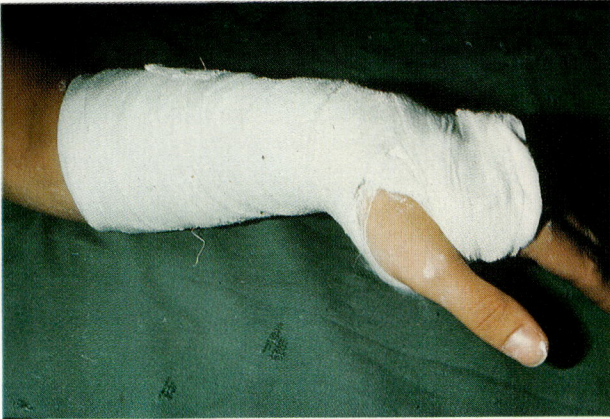

Mr Gray, a 45-year-old crane driver, slipped on a patch of oil at the yard yesterday, sustaining an injury to his left wrist. He was taken immediately to the Accident and Emergency Department of the local hospital. He attends your surgery, requesting 'a certificate'. There has been no communication, as yet, from the hospital.

(a) What sort of certificate might Mr Gray require?
(b) What details would you disclose concerning Mr Gray's condition?
(c) In light of the information given, Mr Gray is unlikely to be fit for work.
  (i) How long is his disability likely to last?
  (ii) For how long would you certify him as unfit?

Presentation 11: Moira Campbell

Moira Campbell is an unmarried bank teller, aged 28 years. For years she's been a martyr to the chronic unsightly skin blemishes pictured. She's tried all sorts of ointments, applications and medications which, at best, only seem to dampen things down.

She has become disillusioned by the inability of the medical profession (she includes yourself as well as the consultant dermatologist in this) to cure her.

She enters your consulting room accompanied by her latest boyfriend (who is not your patient) and shows you the exacerbation of her skin condition.

As you are writing a prescription for her, her boyfriend says, 'Why don't you refer Moira to Mr Meredew – he's cured a friend of mine with his pendulum'. You remember seeing Mr Meredew's advertisement in the local paper yesterday: 'Skin blemishes removed, or your money refunded: specialist in psychokinesis'.

(a) When two adults enter the consulting room, what significance might this hold?
(b) Are you able to comply with the suggestion from Moira's boyfriend?
(c) What emotional reaction commonly accompanies chronic skin disease?

Presentation 12: Sam Brown

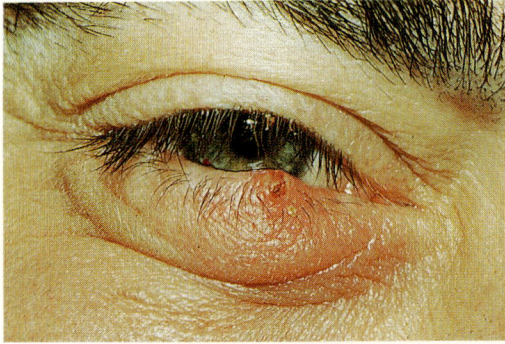

Sam Brown comes yet again, saying in rather an aggressive tone, 'Your treatment's no good, Doc; the irritation and swelling's as bad as last week. Why don't you give me an antibiotic?' He has had this eye condition several times before, together with crops of boils in the past 6 months.

Sam is a joiner, and has the use of only his left eye – the other is completely blind as a result of an injury received in childhood. Married, with two children, he has recently taken on a mortgage for the council house he had rented for the previous 8 years. His wife, Mary, is an anxious inadequate person, frequently bringing their two children with a succession of minor complaints. Toby, the younger child, aged 7, is enuretic.

Sam's mother is also a practice patient. She is an insulin-dependent diabetic with retinopathy.

(a) What is the nature of Sam's problem?
(b) Why might he appear to be so aggressive?
(c) What principles might guide you on managing the situation at this point?

Presentation 13: Bill

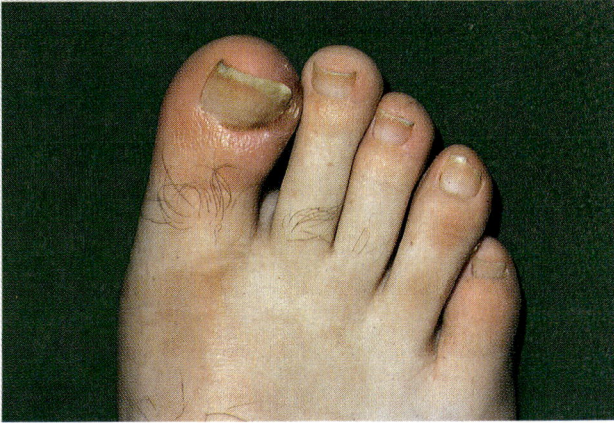

Bill, who plays centre-half (professionally) for his local football team, attended 2 days ago with a recurrence of the foot condition that has plagued him intermittently throughout the season. The practice nurse has been supervising his treatment and when he attends again tonight you find the condition as illustrated. Bill is clearly dissatisfied with progress and says he must play in Saturday's match in 3 days' time. He demands to see a specialist immediately.

(a) What moves might you make?
(b) Might Bill's problem have been prevented – if so, how?
(c) What other health professionals might be involved in Bill's situation?

Presentation 14: Mrs MacAulay

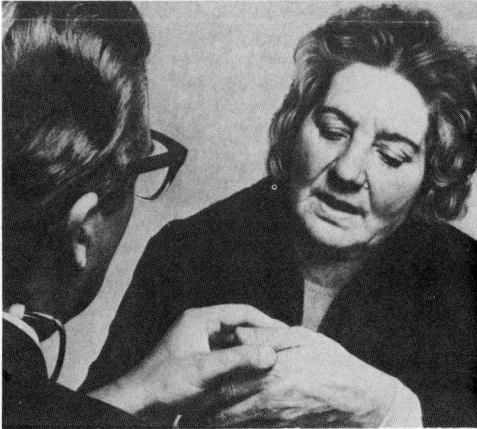

Mrs MacAulay is consulting the senior partner. She says she has a painful swollen area at the base of her left thumb, present for the last few weeks; 'though, of course, I've had it on and off for some time', she continues. 'And I've been that tired lately. And my blood pressure pills haven't done a thing for my breathlessness. I know I'm a bit overweight – it's funny, really: I don't eat a thing – but then I come from 'stout stock'. And the constipation is as bad as ever – though I have to rise two or three times in the night to pass water. 'Course I haven't been the same since the birth of my third boy – he was upside down, you know; it probably accounts for it, his funny ways, and his cousin was just the same at his age – he was upside down too . . .'

You remember that Mrs MacAulay's husband died 4 months ago, and you note she's still dressed in black. Her mother's sister was very crippled with rheumatoid arthritis and was housebound in a wheelchair before she died.

(a) Multiple presentations are not uncommon in general practice. In such a case, where do you begin?
(b) Mrs MacAulay is obviously a garrulous patient. What communication techniques are necessary to ensure the consulting time is put to the best use?
(c) What might be at the root of Mrs MacAulay's 'troubles'?

Presentation 15: John S

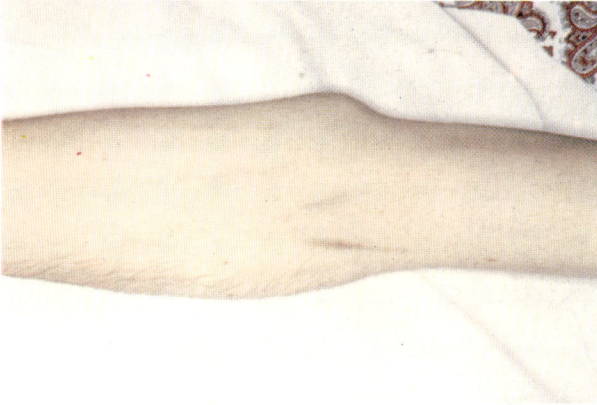

John S, aged 22 years, joins your NHS practice list as an 'allocated patient'. He presents saying, 'I've come for my 13-week line, and my pills – and I need some more Diconals: they're for the headaches'. He does not give a coherent account, but you gather that he was discharged from the army 2 years ago on account of 'dizzy spells' following a head injury. He has apparently been unemployed, and takes 'the tablets' (he produces a bottle of carbamazepine 200 mg tabs). He is of spare build and has a somewhat shifty appearance; physical examination reveals no neurological deficit. You notice thin streaks over the antecubital fossa, along with puncture marks.

(a) What does 'allocated patient' mean?
(b) If he admits to 'mainlining', what further action should you take?
(c) How would you handle his demand for Diconal (dipipanone)?

Presentation 16: Norma G

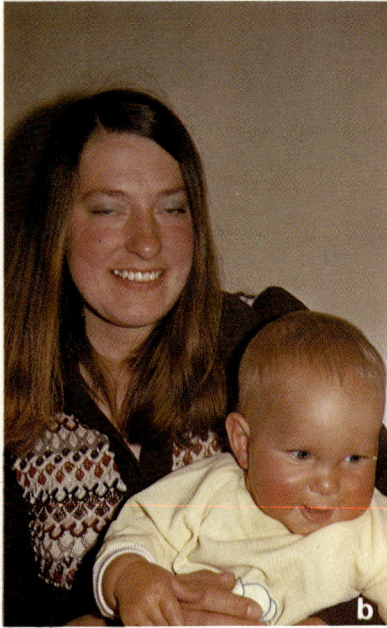

Norma G, 25-year-old mother of Duncan (aged 8 months) attends, with a request for the 'morning-after' pill. She defaulted from follow-up of the oral contraceptive regimen started after her postnatal check, because she had been putting on excessive weight.

(a) What might you do about Norma's request?
(b) What else might you do at this contact?
(c) What follow-up arrangements would you make?

At home

Presentation 17: Sandy

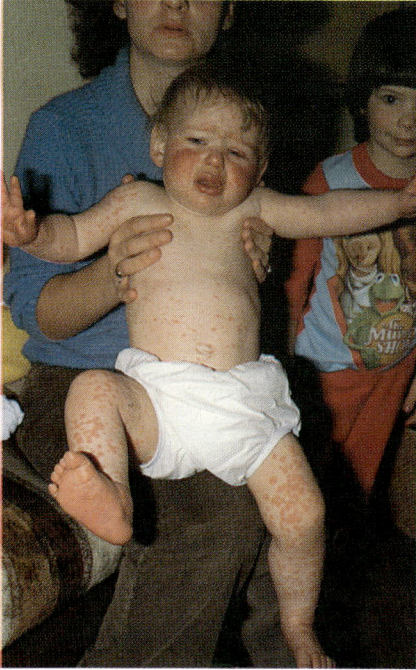

The home visit is to see Sandy, aged 18 months, because his mother is worried he has measles. Over the last 2 days Sandy has not been his usual self, and now he has this blotchy rash on both cheeks. Sandy had his usual lunch today and is up and running about when you visit.

(a) What points in the scenario make a diagnosis of measles unlikely?
(b) If Sandy hasn't got measles, what might be the diagnosis?
(c) What arrangements, if any, might be made for follow-up?
(d) In addition to managing Sandy's situation, what other points might be covered by the doctor at this contact?

Presentation 18: Ethel Smith

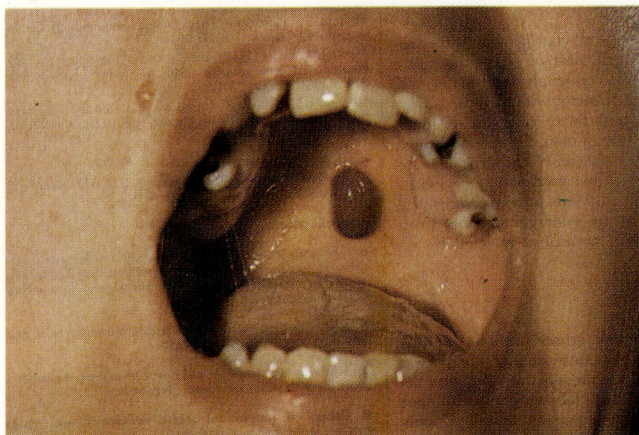

It is your night on call. Miss Ethel Smith telephones at 10.50 p.m. She sounds desperately anxious. 'Oh Doctor,' she exclaims, 'please come at once. It's this terrible thing in my mouth – I think it must be a haemorrhage.' She rings off before you can obtain further details, though you thought her voice had a more 'nasal' quality than was her usual. You remember her as a rather timid spinster now in her fifties, living alone at 31 Ivy Terrace – just down the road.

When you see her at 11 p.m. she tells you that she was having a bit of toast with her glass of milk before retiring to bed and she thinks the toast scratched her palate. Inspection of her mouth reveals the situation shown in the photograph.

(a) Use of emotionally charged words

Some words, in addition to their cognitive meaning, carry an 'emotional charge'. The word 'haemorrhage' (instead of the more neutral 'bleeding') in the transcript of Miss Smith's telephone message may be one example.

(i) Can you give two examples of other such terms which patients (or, more often, their relatives) may use, especially when contacting the doctor?

(ii) What purposes may be served by the use of these terms?

(b) Extent of clinical examination

Of all the possible items in your repertoire of 'thorough physical examination', which would you select as appropriate for Miss Smith's situation in her house at 11 p.m.?

(c) Management

What would you actually do at this contact?

Presentation 19: Mr McLeod

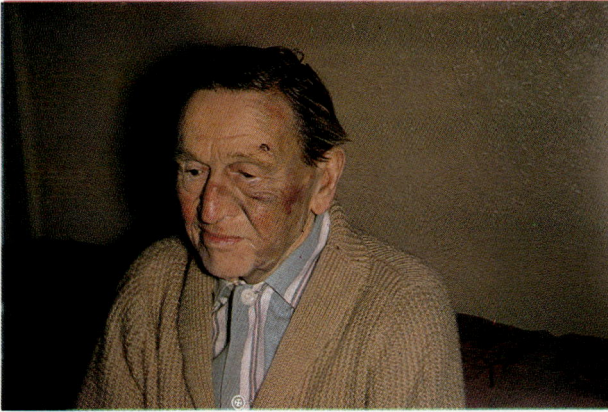

Mr McLeod's neighbour puts in an urgent request because Mr McLeod has had to be brought home having collapsed in the street. You know Mr McLeod as a normally hale and hearty 81 year old who has been living on his own since his wife died 3 years ago.

Your receptionist has interrupted your consulting session to pass on the message: your partner is out on his rounds.

When you call on Mr McLeod, he presents the appearances shown in the photograph.

(a) Assessing urgency of a call

Would you discontinue your consulting to visit in response to this call?

(b) Selective awareness of clinical phenomena

What significant positive and helpful negative clinical phenomena would you look for when you visit Mr McLeod?

(c) Adjusting Mr McLeod's level of dependence

Should you wish to increase Mr McLeod's support, what measures are likely to be open to you?

Presentation 20: Bill Jones

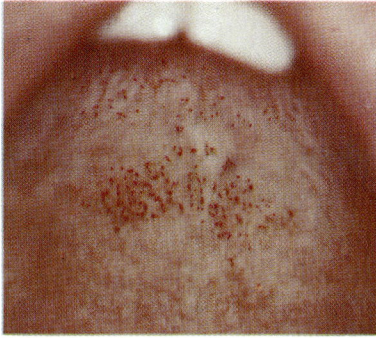

You are on duty for the practice one Saturday afternoon when you receive a telephone call from a Bill Jones. You remember him as a tall, gangling 19-year-old lad whom you don't know well – though you know his parents separated last month. He says he feels unwell, his throat is sore, especially when he swallows, and he requests a home visit from you.

You happen to have another house call in the same street, so you visit Bill. He's on his own and, though he's dressed, he is obviously far from well – pyrexial, with a dirty exudate over both tonsils and enlarged tender cervical glands. You observe the appearance of his palate (*see illustration*). He tells you that his father is due back from a holiday in France tomorrow and that he must go to his work as a barman tonight or he'll lose his job.

(a) List the factors you take into account in planning the management of this episode.
(b) What factors govern the response a principal in NHS general practice makes to requests for a house call?

Presentation 21: Grace P

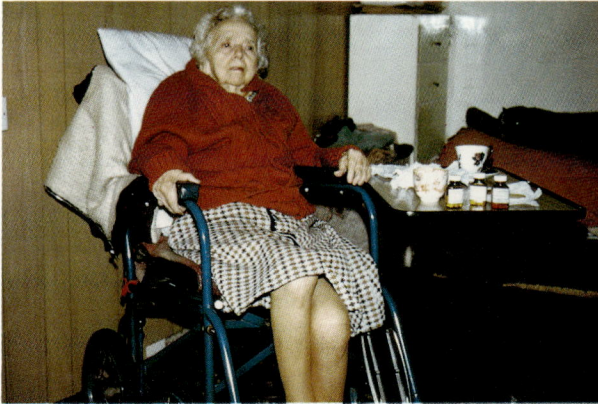

Mrs Grace P, a widow now in her eighties, is pictured in the residential home for the elderly where she has lived for the past 5 years, since the death of her husband. She made a good recovery from a slight stroke 3 years ago, though she is a bit forgetful and rather depressed at times. She now suffers pain and decreased mobility from osteoarthritis of her left hip. At this visit, she complains of increased frequency of micturition. The care assistant tells you that she is in fact often incontinent of urine. Her medication consists of bendrofluazide, piroxicam and nitrazepam, all of which she has been having for many years.

(a) How does Mrs P obtain her supplies of long-term medication?
(b) How is compliance ensured?
(c) As you review Mrs P's problems, what principles guide you in forming plans for her future care?

Presentation 22: Miss Green

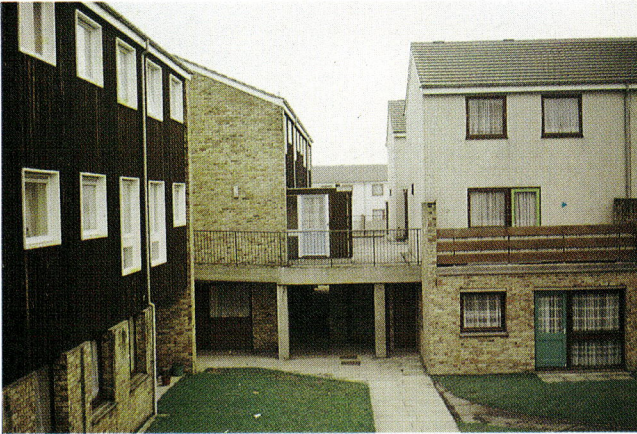

Miss Green, an octogenarian, lives on her own in a first-floor flat in this large housing estate. She is on your periodic visiting list because she is a little confused at times and recently has complained of chronic pain in the left thigh, radiating to the left knee. She is clinically euthyroid, on long-term thyroid replacement therapy. Examination has revealed limitation of all movements in the left hip, especially internal and external rotation. She has difficulty in walking and negotiating stairs, so she finds she now is unable to get to the shops. She is frightened by gangs of noisy youths who use the open area as a nightly meeting place and, with the advent of winter, she has resigned herself to staying indoors.

(a) What is the likely pathogenesis of Miss Green's locomotor impairment?
(b) On the information given, list three of the more pressing of Miss Green's problems.
(c) If, as you anticipate, you find the situation much as before, when will you see her again?

Presentation 23: Walter W

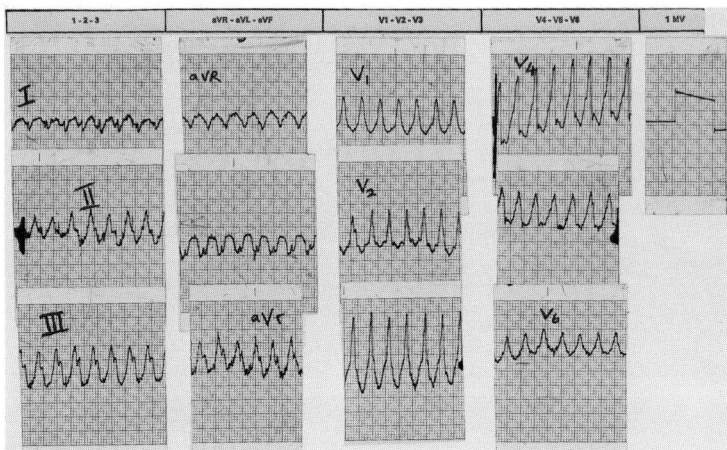

Walter W, a 48-year-old van driver, has been on atenolol for mild hypertension for the past 18 months. His wife 'phones your receptionist from home at 8.30 a.m. saying he has had a bad night with a 'gastric stomach', meaning he has been dizzy and nauseated.

You find Walter in bed, alone in the home, his wife having gone to her work as hairdresser's receptionist. As you greet Walter, he rises to go to the toilet saying he's going to be sick, but on the landing he falls unconscious. He recovers consciousness spontaneously within a couple of minutes and, with difficulty, you get him back to bed. He seems unable to add much to the story and the main objective findings are an auscultated apical heart rate of about 200/min and an unrecordable blood pressure. You have the practice ECG machine in the car and you wire him up for a tracing.

(a) *Physical diagnosis*

   (i) What does his tracing show?
   (ii) Does the absence of chest pain preclude a myocardial infarction?

(b) *Immediate management*

   What factors do you take into account in managing the acute situation?

(c) Practice management issues

    (i) Does the taking of an electrocardiogram attract an item-of-service fee under NHS terms of service?

    (ii) How is the ECG machine provided in general practice?

Presentation 24: Harold Green

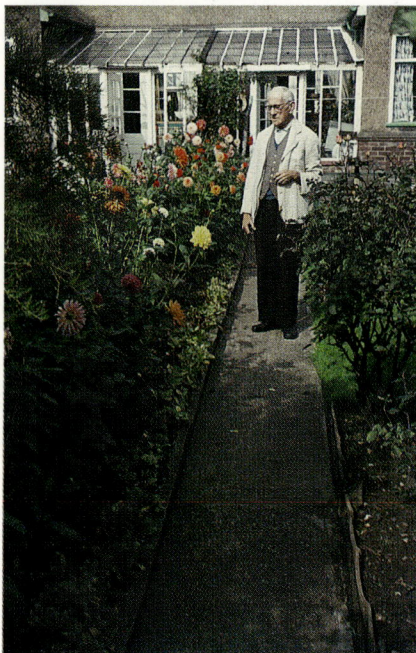

Mr Harold Green, an octogenarian, pictured here in his garden, The Elms, Inchgowrie, remains 'in the pink' on regular maintenance hydroxocobalamin, which he has received ever since his megaloblastic anaemia was diagnosed 10 years previously. The only other item in his past medical record is a brief hospital discharge letter, dated 40 years ago, stating that he had made a good recovery from a partial gastrectomy for duodenal ulcer.

Your visit is partly social – he has offered you a bunch of his prize-winning dahlias – and partly professional, to deliver his prescription for more of his vitamin B_{12}.

(a) Write the prescription for his B_{12}.
(b) How might his B_{12} be administered, and by whom?
(c) What else might his doctor be expected to do?
(d) What significance, if any, might be attached to gifts from patient to doctor?

Presentation 25: Mrs Ambleside

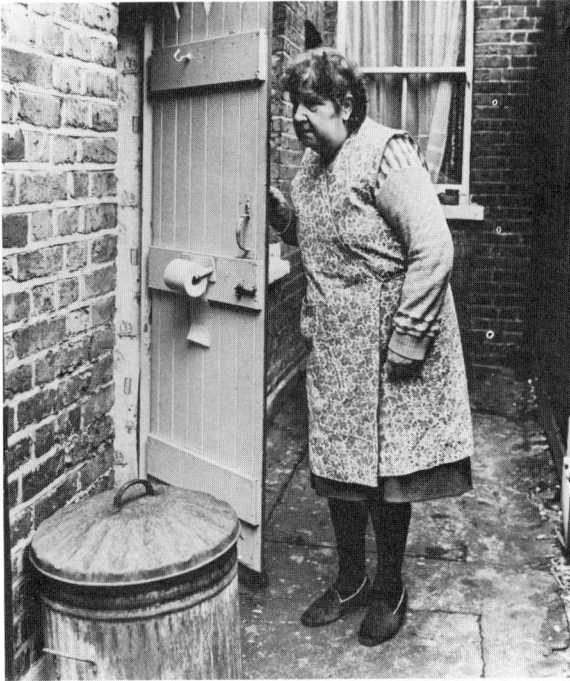

Six months ago Mrs Ambleside, a widow aged 65 years, was discharged from hospital following myocardial infarction complicated by congestive failure. She has become much less mobile since her return, partly because of the swelling of her ankles – she has been prescribed regular maintenance doses of diuretics – and is reduced to wearing slippers (*see illustration*).

She lives alone and her neighbour, who had been looking in every day, is now refusing to visit because Mrs Ambleside is smelly and a bit confused.

(a) From the scenario as pictured and described *above*, indicate the inter-relation of physical, psychological and social factors in Mrs Ambleside's situation.

(b) What roles might the health visitor play in improving Mrs Ambleside's lot?

Presentation 26: Eliz Anderson

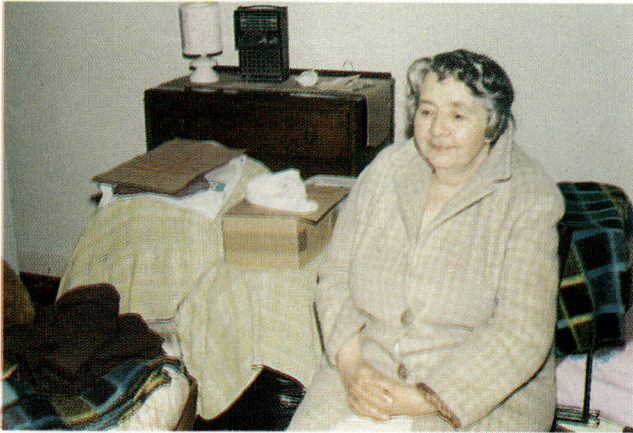

Mrs Eliz Anderson, a widow in her eighties, has just arrived back home from hospital. She had been admitted largely on social grounds, because of a mild bronchitis and diarrhoea precipitated by the antibiotic with which your partner had been treating her prior to admission. She also has a background of diverticular disease and thyroid disease requiring thyroid replacement therapy.

She lives alone in a flat which she has found progressively more difficult to run; prior to admission she had been having the services of a home help twice weekly. Her son is a busy professional man with his own family, living at the other end of the town. Your visit is in response to a request from him, on a Saturday morning. 'She has a letter for you', he says.

(a) In the transfer of care of the elderly across the hospital/community interface, what problems are commonly encountered by the family doctor?
(b) What are the aims you have in making your visit to Mrs Anderson?

Presentation 27: Florence Turner

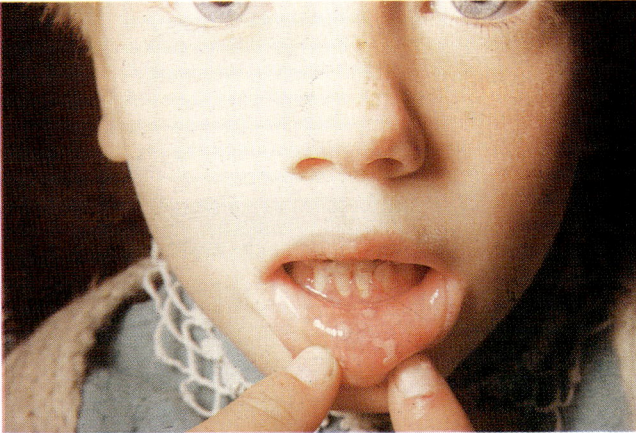

Florence Turner is a 10-year-old schoolgirl, whom you visit at home because she is unwell, running a high temperature and complaining of a sore mouth and a throbbing painful left thumb, all developing in the last 2 days.

(a) If you wished to confirm your clinical diagnosis, what specimens would you take, in what containers, and how would you transmit them to the laboratory?
(b) Florence has a younger sister, Mary, aged 18 months. Mrs Turner asks if you think Mary is at risk of picking up Florence's disease. What would you reply?
(c) Florence is learning to play the clarinet and has an important examination in a week's time. Mrs Turner wonders if Florence will be fit by then. What do you advise?

Presentation 28: Mr Sidon

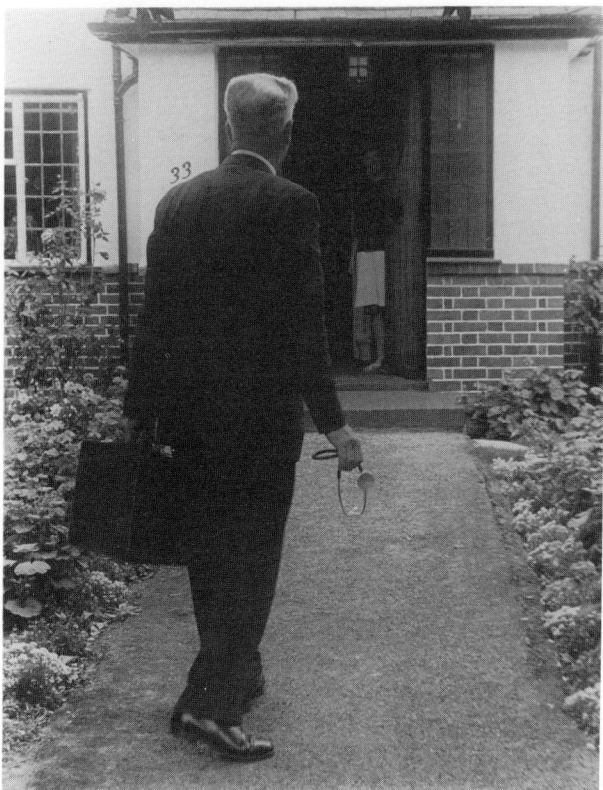

Your visit is in response to an urgent telephone request from Mr
Sidon's wife: 'Oh, Doctor, please come at once – my husband's
collapsed!'. You remember that Mr Sidon, a respiratory cripple
aged 69 years, had been admitted to hospital 3 weeks previously
for transurethral prostatectomy. You were unaware that he is now
back at home, but apparently he was discharged 3 days ago.

You find Mr Sidon slumped in his chair, obviously dead, and
Mrs Sidon (who is not a patient with your practice) is distraught.

(a) Urgent telephone requests and home visits have certain
    characteristics commonly associated with them – identify two
    such characteristics.
(b) What might you take with you on this visit?
(c) What immediate moves might you make at this visit?
(d) If Mrs Sidon should raise the issue of cremation, how might
    you proceed?

Presentation 29: Alex Abel

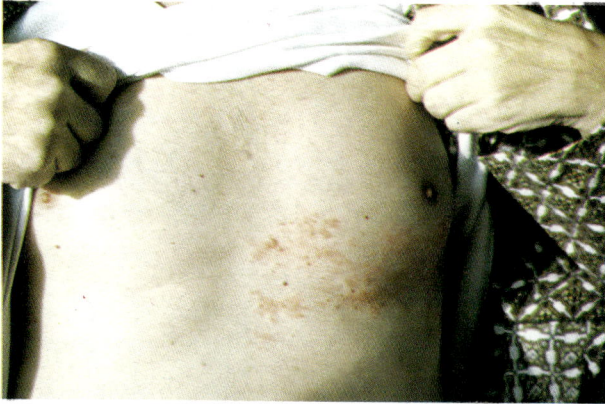

It is 11.30 p.m. one Tuesday night (your night on call). Your visit is in response to Mrs Abel's phoned request – 'It's Alex, my husband. He's been under the weather for the last couple of days and now he seems to have burned himself on the electric blanket.'

Alex, a 60-year-old clerical officer, does not seem ill, but physical examination reveals the appearance in this photograph.

(a) Given that Alex is not seriously ill, what factors might you take into account in assessing his fitness for work?
(b) What 'paper-work', in terms of certificates, prescriptions and other documentation, is likely to be required of you in relation to this visit?

At the surgery premises

Presentation 30: Sister Black and Mr Whyte

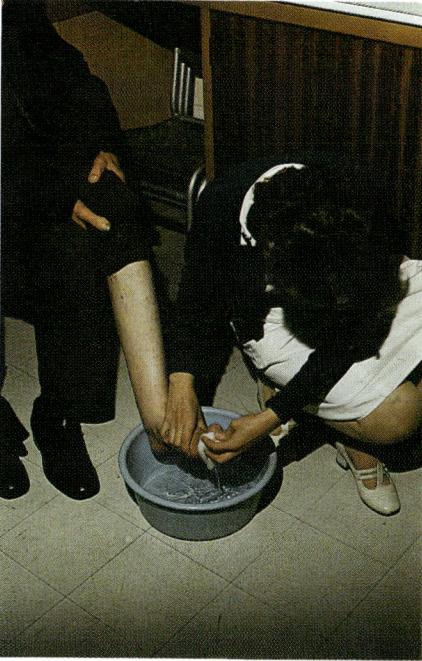

Sister Black is seen in the treatment room washing old Mr Whyte's left foot. He is one of a number of your NHS list of patients who see her without 'bothering' you.

(a) List three conditions which might generate the need being met by Sister Black.
(b) (i) Who employs and pays Sister Black?
    (ii) Who is responsible for her professional actions?
(c) What are the advantages and disadvantages of the different systems of employment of nursing staff in the community?

Presentation 31: Sally and Miss Gray's repeat prescription

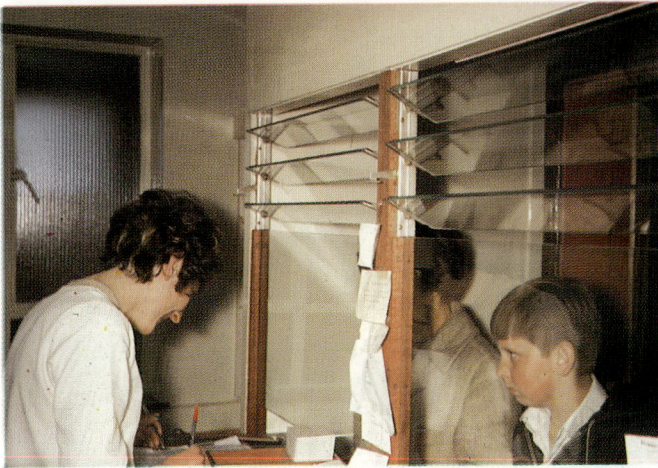

Sally, the practice receptionist, is seen handing over a prescription to Miss Gray's niece, who is collecting it on behalf of her aunt. Miss Gray, a frail octogenarian, is housebound, crippled by senile osteoporosis, and suffers from insomnia. She has sent a written request for a repeat of her non-steroidal anti-inflammatory analgesic, oral calcium preparation and 5 mg nitrazepam tablets (two at night), all of which she has taken regularly for more than 10 years.

(a) Besides handing over prescriptions, what other tasks does Sally perform in her role of receptionist?
(b) What potential problems are inherent in pharmacological solutions to Miss Gray's condition?
(c) What is 'repeat prescribing' and how are repeat prescriptions handled in general practice?

Presentation 32: Gwen

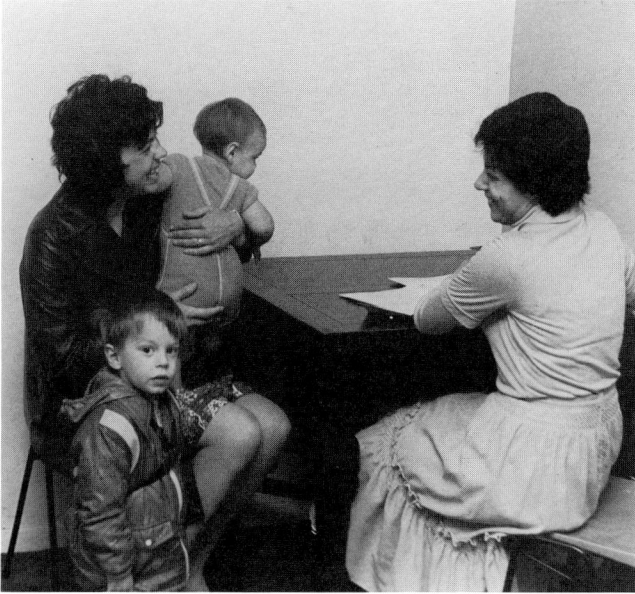

Gwen and her two children, Paul (2) and Barry (1), are pictured attending the well-baby clinic, talking to Mrs Adams, the health visitor.

This is a single-parent family, which has recently joined your NHS practice list, having moved into the practice area.

(a) What items of information relating to each member of the trio would you, as their new family doctor, wish to have?

(b) What arrangements exist in the NHS to ensure the onward transmission of medical records from one general practitioner to another?

Presentation 33: Letter from RS

28th March

Dear Doctor,

I am writing to complain about the obstructive and unsatisfactory behaviour of one of your receptionists on Monday, 27th March.

At approximately noon on that date I phoned your practice seeking urgent advice regarding the apparent collapse of my eight month old daughter. She had displayed a mild constitutional upset associated with teething since the previous evening but was in relatively good spirits. At lunchtime on Monday she refused food, having eaten sparingly all morning, and over a period of some five minutes her skin developed a pronounced pallor and was cold and clammy. She became listless and gradually more unresponsive to her mother.

I found, despite describing the nature of her symptoms and the suddenness of their appearance, that your receptionist failed to appreciate the urgency of the situation and was most unhelpful and obstructive. Even as I spoke my daughter became cyanosed and we took her immediately to hospital.

I know that receptionists can act as an effective 'screen' to protect G.P.s from trivial demands. In this instance, it appears to me that your receptionist was over protective (in a haughtily unpleasant manner) and constituted an impenetrable barrier.

I realise that, with the pressures on general medical practitioners, you can not be readily available for any contingency but I resent having to engage in a harangue with an overbearing receptionist in order to determine the state of your availability.

I would appreciate your comments.

Yours sincerely,

R.S.

In your morning mail you find a letter addressed to you from one of your patients. This family has not been with the practice very long and you barely know them, though you dimly recall your partner saying that your receptionist had had an odd sort of 'phone call from the father a week ago.

(a) Assessing the situation
(i) What does the letter tell you about the writer?
(ii) What additional information, if any, do you need to assess the situation? How would you go about obtaining it?

(b) Responding to the situation

What moves would you make in the light of this letter? Give reasons for your answer.

Presentation 34: Letter from Elizabeth L

11th June

Dear Bill,

You may be approached shortly by Emblem Life Assurance on my behalf.

I told them I was fit and healthy, which is perfectly true, omitting the coeliac condition - would you be a' pet and do the same? I find no one can think straight when some esoteric condition is mentioned and Dr X (Hospital Consultant) did say I was one of the fittest persons for my age he had ever examined.

A lot depends on my acceptance - I'm trying to provide for my retirement, and I can't accept that I should be penalised (perhaps?) for this. I know diabetics can have a rough time and I don't feel in that category at all.

Hope you'll comply, if approached. Am sending this letter for a prescription direct to the Health Centre - going off to Corsica next weekend and need my provisions to take with me.

Hope you're well and have a good holiday when the time comes.

Many thanks.

Yours

E

This is a letter from Mrs Elizabeth L. She lives alone, having been separated from her husband for many years. She is a cheerful extrovert who suffers from gluten enteropathy.

(a) If Emblem Life Assurance approach you with a standard letter requesting information on Mrs L's medical conditions past and present, how will you respond? Discuss relevant issues in the light of the information given above.

(b) What 'provisions' might Mrs L be alluding to in her letter?

Presentation 35: Letter from Mary Seton

Dear Dr X,

I am very sorry I asked you to change my Doctor. I am very very sorry and feel terrible. I was given the wrong advice and in the meantime I am very very hurt and sorry, for I felt terrible. I got on so well with you. I thought there was nobody like you Doctor. I do wish you would give me another chance and take me back. I would be so grateful. I have done nothing but cry. Please forgive me please.

Yours sincerely

Mary Seton

With the morning mail to the practice in which you work as a partner, you receive a hand-written letter addressed to you personally.

You remember Mrs Seton as a demanding, difficult, manipulative patient with a long-suffering husband. You had leaned over backwards in trying to meet her never-ending demands and needs associated with moderately severe chronic obstructive airways disease and psychoneurotic depression. Despite your efforts she decided to change to another general practitioner.

(a) How does a person choose a family doctor and become 'registered' on his NHS list of patients?
(b) If you were to reply to Mrs Seton, what considerations would guide your response?

Presentation 36: Letter from an unknown patient

Begle Farm
Abbeyton, Northington,
England

Dear Sir,

I am writing to you to ask for your help.

For over six years I have suffered a terrible eating disorder compulsive binging, the binging goes on for months and put on an unbelievable amount of weight. I then have to diet for a long long time to remove all the ugly fat I have put on. I have tried hypnosis, seen psychiatrists, diet specialists ate normally with my family all with absolutely no help.

I have now come up with a brilliant idea, I want an intestinal By Pass operation done. I have told my doctor about this and he says if I can come up with information about this operation he will see what he can do. I have read about this in quite a lot of books and do really think that through time this would help my problem enormously. I might still put on weight but it would be at a far, far slower rate and this would be great.

Please could you give me any help on this subject and do you know if they do this at any special units at X and Y [nearby towns] etc.

Thank you

Yours faithfully
CS

In the morning mail you receive, out of the blue, this handwritten letter from someone you have never met and who is not on your NHS list of patients. The address indicates that the writer probably lives in a rural part of the country, and the location is about 100 miles away. You have no idea how or why you have been selected – it might be the result of a talk on 'health and sensible eating' you gave to the local community group last year, but this is pure conjecture on your part.

(a) From your knowledge of the condition referred to in the letter and from the limited information you have, what can you deduce about the writer?
(b) What considerations govern your decisions about a response?
(c) What response might you make?

Discussions on issues selected from the presentations

Introduction to Part II

From each scenario presented in Part I, several issues have been selected for special consideration. They are not necessarily the only possible issues, nor are they always the most important in the management of the given situation. In the second part of this book the issues raised in the scenarios are considered from the standpoint of a general practitioner. The nature of general practice and the relatively small (though rapidly increasing) volume of relevant research mean that many issues are open to a variety of different interpretations, all possibly of equal validity. The views recorded are for the most part based on a wide reading of the relevant literature, modified by the author's personal experience. It is likely that the changing scene in health care will render some of what has been written obsolete and, although efforts have been made to eliminate errors, some mistakes will be included. For these reasons this section should be used by tutors and students as a guide aimed at stimulating critical thinking. Where the reader disagrees with the text, he will gain by discussing with a colleague possible reasons for this divergence of views.

References to the recent literature have deliberately been kept to a minimum and the inclusion of a particular work is dictated by its value as supplementary and complementary teaching on medicine outside hospital.

The following sections on five levels of clinical functioning and 'minor medicine' outline principles which the author has found useful in applying to many of the issues raised in Part I.

Five levels of clinical functioning

Medalie (1965, 1978) identifies a number of levels at which a doctor may function in making decisions.

Level I

The doctor responds to the presentation of a symptom in an automatic way, usually by prescribing a symptomatic remedy. No attempt is made to take the situation to a deeper level. N. Stott (1983) labels this the 'cook-book' approach and cites examples such as cough – soothing linctus, and diarrhoea – kaolin mixture. This 'decerebrate' approach is occasionally forced on the general practitioner by pressure of circumstances. In a context where the orthodox organic medical model may be inapplicable to some 40% of presenting problems, perhaps the cook-book approach is not as harmful as those whose work is in a different setting would have us believe. Nevertheless, this level is not one advocated for regular functioning.

Level II

The response is to apply the orthodox medical model of fitting symptoms and signs to a known pathology which the doctor then attempts to 'cure'. This level of functioning is well suited to the highly selected hospital 'case-material' which forms the basis of orthodox clinical teaching. Wood and Badley (1981) and others have pointed out, however, a shortcoming of this approach in its failure to take adequate account of the concept of disability and handicap, however well it defines the 'impairment'.

Level III

This takes into account more fully the patient's view of his problems and the doctor's proposed solutions. Considerations such as these account for much of the apparent inactivity of more experienced general practitioners in relation to investigative medicine. The decision *not* to take things further is often the result of balancing the likely pay-off, in terms of benefit to the patient, against the likely disturbance the move may create for the patient. This is one example of the *patient-centred* approach.

Level IV

This takes into account actual or potential interactions between the patient's health and the family. It includes physical considerations, such as those immediately at risk to infectious diseases, as well as psychodynamics, for example, those in the alcoholic spouse. Considerations at this level are the norm for most family doctors, whose resulting actions may not always be clear to hospital colleagues: so-called 'social admissions' to hospital are a case in point, where the family doctor may not have spelt out clearly enough that one element in his decision to request admission is to provide temporary respite for the caring relative.

Level V

Considerations at this level take account of what may be happening in the wider community. One example is the doctor's working knowledge of the incidence and prevalence of diseases in his practice area at a given time. Another is the effect on his patient of conditions at work – and *vice versa*.

It is not suggested that the family doctor necessarily works at each of these five levels every time for every patient. Nevertheless, over a period of time which allows him to build up an extensive data base on his patients, their families and his practice, it becomes almost second nature for the experienced general practitioner to think simultaneously in each of these dimensions. What may be more important for the student is to develop a readiness to respond at each of these levels when the well-being of his patient, the practice and himself require such attitudes.

Though these five levels are particularly relevant to the work of general practitioners, the concepts have wide applicability to all situations in which doctors and patients meet in consultation, even when the presentation is apparently only a minor one.

Minor clinical medicine in general practice

Some new entrants to general practice, fresh from hospital experience, are impressed by the apparently relatively minor nature of most diseases confronting them. Others, expecting much 'trivial medicine', are surprised by the range, nature and seriousness of major illness which may contribute up to 30% of the doctor's work. All experience difficulty in adjusting to a very variable situation.

Studies have shown that over 60% of first presentations are minor and usually self-limiting. The proportion decreases with age and with home visiting.

While there is a danger in classifying people, it is helpful to classify presentations so that they may more readily be recognized and appropriately managed. One classification is set out *below*.

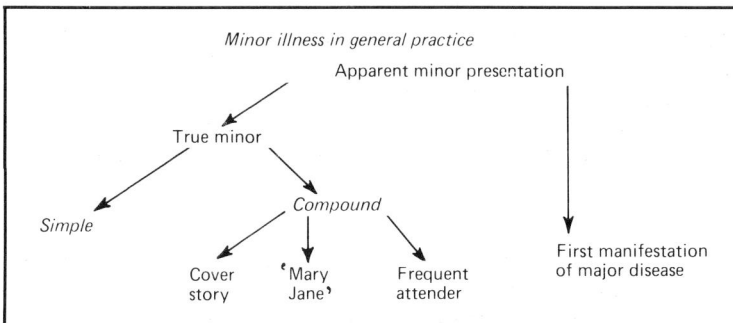

Minor illness in general practice

Single simple

These are the commonest presentations and are illustrated by Part I scenario 7.

In many instances, no drug therapy, beyond simple symptomatic remedies, is required. It is always worthwhile remembering that, though relatively minor in comparison with life-threatening illness, such conditions may cause a disproportionate degree of suffering: psychological significance is often inversely proportional to the degree of seriousness. Thus, a patient suffering severe agony from, say, a perforated duodenal ulcer, is preoccupied with seeking relief from pain, while the patient with 'functional dyspepsia' may be obsessed with fears that the symptoms betoken some dreadful disease like cancer.

Cover story

This type of presentation is much less common. Part I scenario 1 is one illustration and shows three commonly associated features:

(i) The true reason for the consultation concerns a much more 'serious' situation than that first offered.
(ii) The main topic is emotionally charged – embarrassment, guilt or fear are the most usual.
(iii) The topic may be introduced by 'While I'm here . . .' or 'By the way, . . .' or 'I hesitate to bother you with . . .'.

Sometimes it is possible to spot this well in advance, and in all situations where the doctor experiences a sense of puzzlement as to why the patient should be consulting, he should afford the patient the opportunity to bring up other subjects.

'Mary Jane'

This group of presentations is one of a more complex set of problems. They are unlike the 'cover story' because the patient's family and sometimes the unwary doctor are involved in acting out situations not always at a conscious level. The name evinced for this group comes from A.A. Milne's well-known children's verses depicting the doctor (a pompous figure in Shepard's cartoon) attempting to 'cure' Mary Jane, whose real problem appears to be a family unable to cope with her temper tantrums on being given rice pudding.

Once the doctor suspects that the apparent patient is merely the index of a much more disturbed situation, he would do well to enlist the help of others trained in the appropriate skills (understanding and using family dynamics, etc.) such as the health visitor.

Frequent attender

Paul Freeling (1983) has coined the phrase 'recidivist' for the very small number (perhaps less than half a dozen in a practice of 2000) of patients who have in common a very high usage rate of medical (mainly general practitioner) services, a baffling series of presentations – usually not in the text-books – not amenable to treatment, and the habit of persistently reopening issues the doctor has attempted to close. Such patients prove a real threat to themselves because the negative emotional reaction they consciously or unconsciously induce in the doctor may very readily blunt his clinical awareness and acumen. Early signs and symptoms of major disease may then be readily missed.

First presentations of major disease

The main need here is for a sound knowledge of the natural and early history of disease, coupled with a readiness to refer to a specialist colleague, even on slender evidence. One of the important intellectual satisfactions in general practice is the justification of such prompt referral action by subsequent events.

Presentation 1: Minnie W, aged 71 years; a 'while I'm here' presentation of a breast lesion, during a surgery consultation

(a) Constraints and barriers to free communication

Any consideration of communication – a two-way process – must include yourself, as well as the patient and her situation.

The patient, being a spinster with an affliction of a sex-related part of the body, may well be, as she indicates, 'embarrassed'. Such an emotional reaction is potentially 'infectious', so it is important for the doctor to be able to cope with his own, as well as his patient's, feelings. Perhaps this aspect of the consultation might be easier for a lady doctor to handle. The patient has cued the doctor to play this consultation at a relatively 'safe' level and the doctor will feel a strong temptation to collude. After all, the appearances are those of a straightforward eczema in someone known to suffer from this condition. On the other hand (as was indeed the case here), Minnie could be presenting Paget's disease of the breast, a condition which might result in mastectomy or, if left untreated, might lead eventually to her death. Yet the doctor, in the absence of scientifically adequate data, has to cope with his patient and be clinically effective both now and later. He has to balance the probability of the presence of potentially major pathology (and the need to take early definitive action) against the possibility of destroying hope or confronting Minnie with a problem to which she may need time to adjust.

It is likely, however, that Minnie already has her views about the potential seriousness of her condition, as evinced by her help-seeking behaviour.

Is it likely that a self-assured lady of 71 years, who is not a frequent attender, would consult her doctor merely for a cold? The likelihood of the 'cover story' is increased by her 'By the way' presentation. Under these circumstances it would be imperative for the doctor to afford Minnie the opportunity to ventilate her views and her possible fears. Any barrier to such an exchange is more likely to be of the doctor's making.

(b) Sharing information with relatives

What takes place between doctor and patient in the privacy of the consulting room must be protected by confidentiality on the doctor's part. Yet this is not an absolute – there are circumstances when exceptions have to be made. It is important that such decisions to share information with third parties (even close relatives) are made at a conscious level and that the reasons are clear.

In Minnie's situation, the probability of underlying malignancy will press the general practitioner to mobilize early specialist advice and possible action, which means referral to hospital. Mrs McDonald might wish to help at this level. If the doctor has shared his suspicions with Minnie, she might have indicated how far she would wish Mrs McDonald to be involved – there is, after all, the likely prospect of a fairly major operation. If the doctor has not communicated his suspicions to Minnie or discussed possible malignancy at this stage, he may wish to bring a responsible relative along with him through his thinking at an early stage to gain co-operation and even to work through the relatives to help his patient to adjust to a developing situation. In the UK there should be no question, at least at this stage, of medicolegal consideration governing such decisions: this aspect should be adequately covered by the normal requirements of clinical note-taking.

Further reading

CALNAN, J. (1983). *Talking with Patients.* London: William Heinemann Medical Books
FREELING, P. and HARRIS, C.M. (1984). *The Doctor Patient Relationship,* 3rd edn. London: Churchill Livingstone. p.60

Presentation 2: Graham, aged 19 years; aphthous ulcers and other problems presented during a surgery consultation

Graham is an example of the multiple problems/presentations so common in general practice.

(a) Aphthous ulcer

His aphthous ulcer is not a recognized complication of long-term medication with the anticonvulsants named. Grand mal may be associated with biting the tongue or the buccal mucosa; such lesions sometimes take several days to heal during which time they may resemble aphthous ulceration. The situation of the lesion illustrated is not incompatible with such an explanation, but it is typical of idiopathic aphthous ulcer, treatment of which continues to remain on an empirical basis.

(b) Driving

Graham has remained free of fits for over the statutory period (recently reduced from 3 to 2 years) so the way is clear for him to apply for his driving test.

(c) Discontinuing drugs

The way is also clear to discontinue anticonvulsant therapy, though you may wish to try to dissuade Graham from starting to drive until he is off his drugs. From the information given, however, it does not sound as though time is on your side. Whatever the timing, you will wish to withdraw his drugs gradually over a period of several weeks.

Further reading

POND, D.A. and ESPIR, M. (1978). *Medical Aspects of Fitness to Drive*. Ed. A. Raffle. London: Medical Commission on Accident Prevention

Presentation 3: Jim T, in his twenties; a presentation in the consulting room of spots in a patient who shows no strong allegiance to any one doctor

(a) Coming in 'half-way through'

The doctor, faced with the need to assume responsibility for management of an on-going condition hitherto unresponsive to treatment (and likely to remain so), has a number of issues to consider. The patient may have become more critical of the medical profession (and this will include your colleagues), and obvious lines of treatment will have already been explored. On the other hand, the situation presents an opportunity for a new initiative to be taken.

Acne is a notoriously intractable condition, and the general practitioner may well be tempted to refer such a patient to a skin specialist, ostensibly 'for a dermatological opinion'. In Jim's situation this may be justifiable if he raises the question of 'a second (different) opinion', and the aggression inherent in the words 'spots are no better' suggests that Jim should be given the opportunity to discuss his views on the efforts so far made on his behalf. Perhaps a more helpful approach would be to make a further attempt to enable Jim to accept the reality of his relatively minor condition and to overcome whatever might be hindering this (?vanity, girlfriend trouble). The pustular appearance and the fact that he is not at the moment having long-term tetracycline in low dose suggest that this drug may have something to offer.

(b) Intrapractice switches of allegiance

This phenomenon is well known in group practices and appears so far to have attracted little research. Reasons for the occurrence of the switches are probably more complex than may appear. Perhaps the original doctor was not available for follow-up after the original consultation, or the patient's preference could be the factor. Maybe the second doctor colluded, in this intractable problem, in passing the patient to a colleague. One of the principles preserved in the NHS has been the right of the patient to have access to the doctor of his choice. Within a practice, however, too free movement among partners can impede the building up of a broadly based yet detached picture of a patient by any one doctor, and deny the patient the full benefit of personal doctoring necessary for continuity of care. On the other hand, such mobility can sometimes afford both doctor and patient some respite when their interpersonal relationships become stressed.

(c) Letting sleeping dogs lie

Most doctors would probably not raise the issue of Jim's acne. Reasons for this include the relatively minor nature of the affliction, viewed by the doctor, together with the doctor's knowledge that, despite the claims of many, acne remains an intractable condition. A further reason might be the doctor's awareness that his 'spottiness' might be a sensitive issue with Jim, and raising the subject in the absence of a sure cure is likely to be an unproductive move.

The doctor's attitude towards deciding whether to intervene or not may not matter greatly in conditions like acne, but in other health problems, such as alcoholism, for example, the results of the doctor's decision can have far-reaching implications.

Further reading

GRAY, D.J. Pereira (1979). The key to personal care. *Journal of the Royal College of General Practitioners,* **29,** 666–678

Presentation 4: Tommy Adamson, aged 7 years, with septic foot; a Sunday morning consultation

(a) Possible referral

The evidence supports a diagnosis of cellulitis of the foot with lymphangitis. The duration of the condition and Tommy's evident well-being (there is no immediate offer of malaise, and he is ambulant) all suggest a relatively minor disturbance. Tommy's home circumstances sound suitable for continuing his care at general practice level – and his mother's nursing skills could be enlisted to monitor progress. So hospital admission, always a costly 'prescription' by the general practitioner, is not a prime consideration here. If it had been, your choice might depend on the services available: communicable diseases, paediatric medical, paediatric surgical or community hospital are possible options.

Factors influencing the choice might include availability of a bed, professional relationships with local consultants, and preference of parents. Details on how admission to hospital is effected from general practice are set out by Drury (1981).

(b) Further information

Important additional items include Tommy's immunization status and possible personal, or family, history of allergy to penicillin.

(c) General practice management

Of the many considerations only two have been selected:

(i) *Ready availability of drug therapy**
You would normally have available on your surgery premises appropriate drugs to start Tommy's therapeutic regimen, e.g. booster tetanus toxoid, penicillin for parenteral use (together with appropriate syringes and needles) and possible oral penicillins of the 'broad spectrum' type. Such drugs may be obtained under NHS regulations on a 'stock order form'. This aspect of general practice work is appropriately supervised by the practice nurse.

Some pharmaceutical companies make 'starter packs' of antibiotics available to general practitioners free of charge for use in situations such as Tommy presents. If, for any reason, the drugs you wish are not immediately available on the surgery premises, or if you wish to manage Tommy's case in a more leisurely fashion, you might initiate his therapy by issuing a prescription to be dispensed by the local retail pharmacist who is obliged under NHS regulations to be available 'out of hours', usually by rota. If you wish to ensure the immediate provision of antibiotic therapy under NHS regulations, you could mark the NHS prescription form 'Urgent'.

(ii) *Follow-up arrangements*
It would seem reasonable to have Tommy rest his foot, though bed rest is not indicated. This means that he will be off school (probably for a week). You might request his parents to bring Tommy back to see you on Tuesday next, or to contact you sooner if they are worried. If you did not adopt this 'low profile' approach but were to initiate antibiotic therapy by

---

* The special situation of dispensing practices is not considered here.

parenteral injection, the parents might be justified in their expectation of a follow-up visit the following day – and Monday is usually a Bad Day in general practice (and Tommy lives at a distance). You might delegate the further management to your nursing Sister (or District Nurse) choosing to inflict a further series of injections on Tommy, but Sister's time could probably be put to better advantage in nursing other practice patients, and Tommy would prefer oral therapy.

Local dressings are probably not required

Further reading

DRURY, M. (1981). *The Medical Secretary's and Receptionist's Handbook,* 4th edn. London: Baillière Tindall

Presentation 5: Jimmy, aged 14 years; a left-sided facial swelling

(a) Differential diagnosis

Common causes of a localized, slightly painful, swelling of sudden onset in a previously well pubescent boy include mumps and lymphadenitis, the commonest cause of which in this instance is infection from a carious tooth. Local inspection will quickly resolve the issue, which is further clarified should there be other patients in the practice suffering from 'epidemic parotitis' (which need be neither 'epidemic' nor 'parotitis'!).

(b) Drug treatment

(i) If (as was the case with Jimmy) the diagnosis is one of mumps, most general practitioners would probably suggest analgesics such as aspirin or paracetamol, to be purchased as home remedies, and would not prescribe them unless Jimmy's father were to make an issue of it. ('So you're not giving him anything then – is that it?') Some might argue the case for attempting to prevent the relatively uncommon complication of mumps orchitis, especially at puberty, by giving oral prednisolone. The evidence to support such a move is inadequate.

(ii) Were a prescription to be given, at the time of writing (1984) Jimmy would be entitled to obtain his medication free of charge because he is under 16 years of age.

(c) Level IV considerations – the family

In considering this issue, we have progressed from the first level ('submandibular swelling'), past the second ('mumps') and the third (mumps affecting Jimmy, a pubescent boy), to consider possible implications for the family (*see p.51 for further discussion of the concept of levels of clinical activity*). Most doctors would say, 'Sorry, there isn't anything I can do about Marie – besides, the infection has probably taken place by now. Anyway, mumps is not a serious disease as a rule and, if she does get it, then that's one disease less to worry about in future.'

(d) Level V considerations – society

(i) The family doctor is concerned not only with individual patients but also with families – and with the society in which he works. At a simple level, this could merely be his collection of patients – the practice population. Consideration of Jimmy's case in this light raises questions of the general practitioner's statutory duties in relation to certain infectious diseases. Mumps is not a notifiable disease; if it were, the appropriate form would have to be filled in and sent to the authorized medical officer appointed by the Health Authority for monitoring communicable diseases.

(ii) Exclusion from school, though not mandatory in most schools, is customary, until the swelling (and malaise, if any) has subsided – usually within 1 week.

Further reading

BENNISON, J. and MARINKER, M. (1982). Changes in facial appearance. In *Practice – a Handbook of Primary Medical Care*. Eds. J. Cormack, M. Marinker and D. Morrell. London: Kluwer Medical. Ch.3.14

Presentation 6: Harry Smith, a 65-year-old
clerk with a right preauricular swelling

(a) High- and low-frequency users of medical services

On average, each person in the UK makes use of his general practitioner just under four times in a year. There is a wide range, with greater frequencies at the age extremes, and women consult more frequently than men. There is an interesting, largely unexplained U.K. geographical distribution, with higher frequencies in the north than in the south. Harry appears to be a singularly low user. So when such a patient consults, the possibility should be entertained that the reason for consulting is pressing and this may denote the presentation of major illness, considered to be 'serious' by the patient and/or his family. This can be a signal to the doctor to be selectively aware for the presence of such pathology and to be especially careful in his use and non-use of 'reassurance'.

(b) Enlisting specialist help

Considering the limited clinical information, the doctor would be justified in making a tentative diagnosis of mixed tumour of the parotid salivary gland. Such an hypothesis needs histological confirmation, involving biopsy. Early referral to a general surgeon is indicated.

(c) Talking to the patient

As in the case of Minnie W (*see p.56*), the issues inherent in this consultation include

(i) the doctor's diagnostic uncertainty and the dilemma of his need for positive action, despite this uncertainty
(ii) consideration of Harry's help-seeking behaviour
(iii) a willingness to bring Harry into the decision-making concerning management. This might be particularly relevant in Harry's situation because, unlike Minnie, there are the additional variables of fitness for work and a spouse to consider.

Useful contributions the doctor might make at this consultation after examining Harry include, 'I know you don't *know* what this is, but I wonder what you or your wife thought about it – why has she nagged you about it?'. And, if Harry confesses to a fear of cancer, 'Well, I can't be certain at this early stage – but let's find out'.

Further reading

COURTENAY, M.J.F., CURWÉN, M. P. *et al.* (1974). Frequent attendance in a family practice. *Journal of the Royal College of General Practitioners*, **24**, 251–261

Presentation 7: Robert, an AA patrolman in his forties, presenting with 'chilblains'

(a) Chilblains

This condition is a good example of one of the 'single minor' presentations seen in general practice, though rarely in hospital. It is probably more prevalent in the community than its relative infrequency in general practice would indicate (perhaps two a year in a practice of 2000). The condition is a vasculitis triggered by cold and there appears to be a personal idiosyncracy – some people exposed to the same physical conditions do not develop the painful, itchy–burning erythematous blotches on the extremities, usually the toes (though hands may be affected). The lesions usually appear in response to cold weather and may occasionally, as here, be associated with impaired nutrition of the skin, which may break down. Healing is usually complete and the lesions disappear spontaneously provided due attention is paid to keeping the extremities warm.

(b) Selective history, examination and investigation

Other forms of peripheral vascular disease may be considered in the differential diagnosis of severe chilblains, so it is appropriate to enquire about Robert's smoking habits, possible undue thirst, weight loss and general health. His peripheral pulses at femoral, popliteal, posterior tibial and dorsalis pedis levels should be ascertained.

(c) Advice

In the light of the above, Robert should be advised to purchase fur-lined boots, roomy enough to take two pairs of socks if need be. He needs to pay particular attention to hygiene, washing and drying his feet and applying talc. He might be encouraged to discuss with his employer ways of avoiding exposure to extremes of cold, while still remaining at work, in the knowledge that you will support him to the hilt with medical certificates if necessary.

(d) Drugs

Despite laboratory evidence of improvements in peripheral blood flow following the oral administration of various vasodilators, many clinicians regard such preparations as of little value (Tring, 1977). Claims have been made for corticosteroids, intravenous calcium and a variety of other agents, but it seems likely that drug therapy has little to offer the chilblain-sufferer.

Further reading

TRING, F.C. (1977). Chilblains. *Nursing Times,* **173,** 1752–1753

Presentation 8: Joanna B, aged 21 years; seen in the consulting room with probable allergy and possible pregnancy

(a) Making a start

Joanna is another multiple presentation. To her, perhaps the more pressing issue – interestingly, the one she has presented second – is the question of possible pregnancy. It would be logical, therefore, to take this one first. If this is a first pregnancy, diagnosis at 5–10 weeks should be relatively straightforward. If her contraceptive status is in doubt (she may have been obtaining supplies of the pill from a Family Planning Clinic), specific enquiry should clear the issue. Collateral suggestive symptoms – morning sickness, increased frequency of micturition, a feeling of fullness in the breasts – may support objective breast changes such as Montgomery's tubercles and increase in pigmentation of the areolae. Some general practitioners keep supplies of 'DIY' pregnancy tests such as 'Gravindex' and at this stage an opportunistic sample of urine taken at this consultation is likely to give a positive result. Robinson and Barber (1977) present a useful summary of the predictive value of each of the phenomena mentioned. If pregnancy is confirmed, it is always worthwhile giving the patient an opportunity to share her feelings about the situation and to take them into account in further decision-making. You will also remember to request her to sign the appropriate form which, under NHS regulations, will allow you to claim such fees as may be due to you.

(b) Drugs and pregnancy

Since the Thalidomide disaster, the occurrence of pregnancy will always raise doubts, at least in the patient's mind if not in the doctor's, about the advisability of any drug therapy.

Joanna may be suffering from angio-oedema, which is a potentially fatal condition, with the risk of glottal oedema – and now she is exhibiting involvement of oral tissues. However, her antihistamine in its present dose has not been effective. It might be justifiable to discontinue all drug therapy for the duration of pregnancy, and to back this move with giving her a supply of adrenaline in injectable form, combined with an instruction to contact the practice if her tongue becomes involved. You might also wish to give her a personal card to carry with her, indicating that she suffers from angio-oedema. Steroid therapy, oral or parenteral, is probably contraindicated on the evidence given.

(c) Prescription charges

Sufferers from allergy are not eligible for special exemption from prescription charges, though it might prove cheaper for a person on long-term drug therapy for a condition such as angio-oedema to apply for a prepaid 'season ticket' issued by the Family Practitioner service of the local Health Authority.

If Joanna is pregnant, however, this becomes a non-issue, because at the time of writing (1984) pregnant women are automatically exempt from prescription charges.

Further reading

ROBINSON, E.H. and BARBER, J.H. (1977). Early diagnosis of pregnancy in general practice. *Journal of the Royal College of General Practitioners*, **27**, 335–338

Presentation 9: Terence Wilton, aged 45 years; the oil executive with the painful anal region

(a) Examination

Mr Wilton is suffering from fissure-in-ano. He may also have piles, but you would be a cruel doctor to attempt to take matters further at this consultation without applying a local anaesthetic. Further examination may safely be deferred until he has returned from his business trip.

Acute fissures usually heal spontaneously: in the meantime the pain may be eased by the application, twice daily, of a local anaesthetic ointment, for a period of a week to 10 days. Longer courses may increase the risk of provoking a local sensitivity reaction. Mr Wilton should be advised to avoid constipation by increasing his fluid intake – purgatives are best avoided.

(b) Practice equipment

Unlike his hospital consultant colleague, the NHS principal in general practice is not a 'health service employee' – he is an 'independent contractor'. As such he is a self-employed business-man and provides his own equipment. His remuneration is adjusted at national level to take this item into account, and he may claim expenses against income tax. Disposable syringes and needles are one exception to the generalizations made here. Used plastic gloves and soiled dressings are removed by arrangement with the local authority and should be incinerated.

(c) Travel abroad

International statutory inoculation requirements for foreign travel have become less stringent in recent years, partly due to the successful eradication of smallpox. Gambia still requires a valid certificate for yellow fever inoculation: once performed, cover lasts for up to 10 years. Let's hope Mr Wilton is already in possession of a valid certificate, because inoculation is performed only at duly authorized centres, and usually in batches: it might therefore be very difficult to lay this on at short notice. Most travel agents have a professional duty to keep up to date with a changing scene. General practitioners are notified periodically through Health Department circulars, and one enterprising 'free through the letter box' weekly contains an insert providing at a glance information on health requirements for travel to most countries of the world.

The NHS general practitioner has no obligation to provide such medicines as Mr Wilton is demanding; he may be encouraged to purchase over-the-counter prophylactics for travellers' diarrhoea, though evidence of their efficacy is weak.

Further reading

WALKER, E. and WILLIAMS, G. (1983). *ABC of healthy travel*. London: British Medical Association

Presentation 10: Mr Gray, aged 45 years; a crane driver with his wrist in a plaster-of-Paris cast, seen in the consulting room

Certificates

(a) Doctors providing general medical services under the NHS Acts are required to give their patients, free of charge, statements required under the Social Security Acts. Mr Gray, as an insured person, is required to support his claim for benefit by such a statement once his spell of incapacity for work has exceeded 7 days. His story and a plaster cast of the type he has suggest that he has sustained a Colles' fracture (a plaster cast for fractured scaphoid might be expected to extend further up the thumb to the level of the interphalangeal joint). He is likely to be unfit for his work for more than a week, so, although strictly speaking he does not require a *doctor's* certificate until a further 5 days have elapsed, most general practitioners would issue a Form Med 3 (Medical Evidence for Social Security) at this consultation; and some would say the doctor who saw Mr Gray at A & E would have avoided Mr Gray's unnecessary attendance at your surgery by giving him his Form Med 3 yesterday.

(b) The diagnosis of the disorder must be stated on Form Med 3 as precisely as possible. Since the certificate is being given in confidence to Mr Gray, in the first instance, this should be a straightforward statement such as 'Injury to wrist – possible Colles' fracture'. There are occasions when, for the patient's well-being, it might be better to give an imprecise statement of diagnosis. If the doctor were to do this, he should then inform the appropriate Medical Officer of the DHSS of the facts using a special form (Form Med 6) for this purpose.

Since Mr Gray sustained his injury at work, he may be entitled to claim injury benefit, and if he is left with a significant permanent disability he may eventually be eligible for an award under the Workman's Compensation Acts. For these reasons, the doctor issuing Mr Gray's certificate should endorse it 'sustained at work'. Mr Gray may also wish to obtain a 'private certificate' for personal insurance purposes. He would be responsible for payment of the fee the doctor is entitled to charge in such a case. The British Medical Association issues guidelines concerning the level of such fees from time to time.

(c) Fitness for work

(i) In the absence of full information from the hospital you are not in a position to answer the questions regarding duration of disability. However, management at this consultation requires you to make an informed guess. If he has sustained a Colles' fracture then, considering the nature of his work, the doctor would be justified in thinking in terms of some 4–6 weeks' incapacity.

(ii) There is usually some element of doubt about duration of incapacity. Furthermore, most general practitioners would wish to keep an eye on Mr Gray's progress, even though he may have been given a follow-up appointment at a hospital fracture clinic. For these reasons, although it is open to the NHS general practitioner to give a statement of incapacity of up to 6 months' duration straight away, most doctors would indicate a spell of 2 or 4 weeks in Mr Gray's situation.

Further reading

DHSS (1983). *Medical Evidence for Social Security and Statutory Sick Pay Purposes*. London: DHSS

Presentation 11: Moira Campbell, aged 28 years, accompanied by her boyfriend, expressing dissatisfaction with the progress of her chronic skin condition

(a) Two adults at a consultation

This phenomenon is always significant. At a simple level, the explanation may be in the problem which may involve and be seen to involve each of the parties – for example, an elderly couple requesting vaccination against influenza. The phenomenon may relate to physical infirmity, as when a frail or disabled patient is helped into the consulting room.

Often, however, the presence of two adults carries psychological undertones, perhaps of pressure to be exerted on the doctor (as in the given situation) to ensure a second (and possibly different) opinion. It may be associated with feelings of dissatisfaction on the part of patient and/or relative. Again it may simply be the expression of a patient's feelings of insecurity in the presence of doctors.

It is always worth the doctor's while attempting to diagnose the emotional situation. In general practice it is as important to diagnose fear as it is to diagnose fever, anger as well as angina, and envy as well as eczema!

(b) Referral to medically unqualified colleagues

In the past, the situation was relatively simple and the answer to Moira's boyfriend would be a firm 'No'. Most family doctors would probably still decline to fall in with the suggestion, but the situation has changed. It is now accepted, for example, that where the doctor decides that it is in the best interests of his patient to be referred to a social worker or chiropodist, such referral is ethically acceptable. In the case of Mr Meredew, however, where financial exploitation of the patient is a possibility, referral could lay the doctor open to a charge of 'unprofessional conduct'. Even here, however, the situation is changing, as exemplified by the wider acceptance of acupuncture. Some doctors, faced with the challenge posed by Moira's boyfriend, might resolve the issue by a passive acceptance, tempered by a desire not to obliterate the hopes Moira and her boyfriend might entertain regarding the 'new cure'. Such a response would not commit the doctor to active referral, but would not prevent Moira from taking this initiative should she so wish.

(c) Emotional concomitants of chronic skin disease

Chronic diseases such as psoriasis (as here) and certain forms of eczema are usually accompanied by a feeling, in the patient, of contamination and 'dirtiness'. Reactions of the lay public as, for example, in crowded buses or lifts, sometimes reinforce such negative feelings. Part of the doctor's job in providing continuity of care to such sufferers is to show acceptance of the patient as a person: it sometimes helps to afford such patients opportunities to ventilate their feelings on this score. Such support may be afforded the patient in other ways; for example, membership of the Psoriasis Association.

Further reading

BRITISH MEDICAL ASSOCIATION (1984). *BMA Handbook on Medical Ethics*. London: British Medical Association

Presentation 12: Sam Brown, seen with an uncomfortable lesion of the left lower eyelid

(a) Sam's problem

From the evidence, Sam appears to be suffering from a simple hordoleum, or stye, a self-limiting minor infection of the hair follicle of an eyelash. Since Sam has been through this before he is likely to know this, so the 'problem' is not just his stye. It appears to be a series of fears related to his stye and conditioned by his past experience, present situation and family circumstances. Possible relevant factors include

(i) fear (irrational) that his vision, already compromised, might be affected and with it his livelihood
(ii) displacement of emotion from a probable disturbed marital/ family relationship
(iii) worry about possible inheritance of his mother's trouble.

(b) Aggressive patients

The factors mentioned above, combined with an element of dissatisfaction with your past therapeutic endeavours, may find their expression in truculence and aggressive behaviour.

(c) Management of Sam and his problem

On purely clinical grounds, further bacteriological examination of his stye is not indicated – the clinical evidence is sufficient for you to make a firm diagnosis of a self-limiting condition, and material suitable for helpful laboratory examination is unlikely to be obtainable by swab. His family history of diabetes mellitus and his past history of recent recurring skin infections might prompt an on-the-spot check for glycosuria; this should be preceded by affording Sam an opportunity to ventilate his grievances. One useful technique to open up this area is simple 'confrontation', in terms such as, 'Well, Sam, as you know you have a nasty stye, but it's coming on slow but sure. You seem pretty angry with me . . . ?'

Normally, antibiotic therapy has little part to play in the management of styes – spoon bathing is probably as useful as anything. However, faced with an angry patient who may well expect antibiotics, and in whom spoon bathing has not been associated with improvement at follow-up, if the doctor were to prescribe an antibiotic, it should be one which is effective against *Staphylococcus aureus*.

Further reading

JACKSON, C.R.S. (1975). *The Eye in General Practice*, 7th edn. London: Churchill Livingstone

Presentation 13: Bill, a professional footballer, is reviewed after a short course of treatment for his painful toe

(a) Bill's toe

Understandably, Bill is frustrated by the slow natural history of an in-growing toenail and at its disastrous interference with his professional life. The first point to tackle is this frustration and a sympathetic approach is called for, in allowing him to give vent to his feelings. The second point is a professional reappraisal of his physical condition. The evidence suggests that the time has come for surgical intervention. Various procedures are in vogue; most involve the resection of nail bed, either partial or complete. While this operation can be carried out, under ring block, in the treatment room, many general practitioners have access to a 'minor-ops' service given by local surgical colleagues: on the principle that it does not make sense 'to keep a dog and bark yourself', reinforced by the patient's expressed wish ('I wish to see a specialist'), most general practitioners would refer Bill promptly, probably to Accident and Emergency, though other arrangements may be made in different parts of the UK.

In Bill's case it would seem fair to him, and to your surgical colleague, to point out that whatever moves are made, he is unfit for Saturday's game and will probably miss out on training and playing for the next 3 weeks. Accordingly, you could issue him with a medical certificate (Form Med 3).

(b) Prevention

It is suggested that cutting the toe nail horizontally (as here) and resecting a small V-shaped area in the middle of the upper edge are useful prophylactic measures. Perhaps Bill needs also to pay particular attention to his football boots and to ensure that, as with his other footware, there is sufficient room to prevent crowding of toes. He will need to pay particular attention to foot hygiene.

(c) Other health professionals

Bill is already having professional care from the practice nurse, under your direction, and you are seriously considering referral to a consultant surgeon – either a general surgeon or the consultant in charge of Accident and Emergency (often an orthopaedic surgeon). Bill probably has ready access to a professional physiotherapist through his football team, which may even have its own medical adviser, and both may have been consulted. Another person from whom Bill may already have sought advice is the chiropodist. Many such professionals run a private practice, or may be in contract with the Health Authorities to provide services under the NHS: these services tend to be concentrated on meeting the needs of the elderly, so if Bill has consulted a chiropodist he is likely to have done this privately.

Further reading

KNOX, J.D.E. and CORMACK, J.J.C. (1982). Ankle and foot problems. In *Practice – a Handbook of Primary Medical Care.* Eds. J. Cormack, M. Marinker and D. Morrell. London: Kluwer Medical. Ch. 3.69

Presentation 14: Mrs MacAulay, who does not stop talking, bombards the doctor with numerous complaints

(a) Multiple presentations

The new entrant to general practice sometimes feels keenly the absence of a clinical orientation to the consultation outside a specialty clinic. If only Mrs MacAulay were being seen by the rheumatic clinic doctor! He could then focus solely on the probably generalized osteoarthrosis. But within the first 2 minutes, the general practitioner is confronted by additional possibilities of depression ('reactive' as part of bereavement), hypertension, obesity, poor drug compliance, hypothyroidism, cystitis, uteric prolapse (? is she also due for a cervical smear), and hints of behavioural disorders (including the epilepsies) in her son – and all to be sorted out within 6 minutes if studies of general practice are to be believed (Balint and Norrell, 1973)!

Fortunately, the general practitioner does not have to sort everything out at once – he has, and can create, opportunities over a period of time in which to operate. Since people often put first those things they regard as important, the doctor can make a start with the first of Mrs MacAulay's symptoms, the discomfort at the base of the thumb, and make a mental note to pursue other elements in her complex presentation later.

(b) The garrulous patient

The doctor needs information, pieced together in an orderly fashion, from which he may construct a picture to be assessed professionally. So, while encouraging a flow of talk by facilitating techniques such as appearing to listen with interest, he needs to use methods to direct the flow into areas which he sees as having potential interest. He may on occasion have to break the flow, by sudden questions combined with shifts of posture, and re-establish the initiative to control the interview. Subjecting the patient to physical examination is one way of regaining control.

(c) Making sense of 'noise'

When so much is going on in a consultation, there is a danger of missing the important cue because of a low 'signal-to-noise' ratio. However, sometimes it is not the individual complaints that are significant, so much as the overall presentation. Mrs MacAulay's multiplicity of symptoms may be the result of hypochondriasis, itself an expression of her personality, or possibly her bereavement is merging into a reactive depressive illness. A knowledge of Mrs MacAuley before her bereavement might be of diagnostic help. This is one example of the advantages of working with a defined population over a period of time – an advantage not often shared by hospital colleagues.

Further reading

BALINT, E. and NORRELL, J.S. (Ed.) (1973). *Six Minutes for the Patient: Interactions in General Practice Consultation.* Mind and Medicine Monographs, No.23. London: Tavistock Publications
ENELOW, A.J. and SWISHER, S.N. (1972). *Interviewing and Patient Care.* London: Oxford University Press. Ch.4

Presentation 15: John S, aged 22 years; an 'allocated patient', requesting dipipanone and a sickness certificate

(a) 'Allocated patients'

An allocated patient is one for whom you are required to provide general medical services. He is likely to have been removed from his previous doctor's NHS list of patients because of unacceptable behaviour (in John's case it was aggressive behaviour to practice staff). Should the patient be unable to find another doctor, the NHS administration responsible for primary care services will undertake the task of finding a new doctor for such a patient.

(b) Notification

There is enough information in scenario 15 to raise a suspicion of abuse of dangerous drugs under Class A of the Misuse of Drugs Act 1971 (*British National Formulary*, 1984). The doctor should attempt to confirm his suspicion, and he is required by the Misuse of Drugs Regulations 1973 and by his terms of service to check whether or not his patient has been registered as an addict. This check can be made by telephoning the appropriate authority, who, to preserve confidentiality, will return the call with the required information, usually within minutes. If the suspect's name is not on the Index, notification must be made in writing within 7 days of the doctor's first becoming aware that his patient may be an addict.

(c) Prescribing controlled drugs for addicts or suspected addicts

In John's case, the doctor needs urgently to check the situation with his previous doctor (*see p.107*). In the meantime he should prescribe only the carbamazepine. There is no clinical evidence of a condition requiring Diconal (dipipanone), which is a preparation that finds a ready market in the illicit drug scene. There may be a case for rapid referral of the patient to the local centre staffed by doctors specially licensed by the Home Secretary to prescribe Class A drugs for addicts.

Further reading

British National Formulary, No.8 (1984). London: British Medical Association and The Pharmaceutical Society of Great Britain. pp. 25–27

Lancet (1984). Notes and News. Licensing restriction for prescription of dipipanone (Diconal). *Lancet*, **i**, 354

Presentation 16: Norma G, aged 25 years,
requesting the 'morning-after' pill

(a) Postcoital contraception

As a first move it is worth trying to assess the risk of pregnancy: after mid-cycle this may be of the order of 20%. In Norma's case, she was unable to give a clear indication because the periods had been very irregular since she stopped taking the pill 3 months ago. She was very anxious to avoid a further pregnancy as she found Duncan 'a bit of a handful'.

At this point Norma could be given an opportunity to express her views on where she considers family planning to end and abortion to begin. There is general agreement that implantation is the event which separates the two, and the 'morning-after' pill is believed to act by preventing implantation.

Among the options are the Juzpe method – 500 μg levonorgestrel + 100 μg ethinyloestradiol (2 tabs Eugynon 50) given stat and repeated in 12 hours. About one in three women so treated will experience a fair degree of nausea and possibly vomiting. The method is considered to be highly (though not absolutely) effective and safe. There is, however, a risk of ectopic pregnancy; for this reason, Norma was advised to let the doctor know if she experienced lower abdominal pain.

(b) Further action at the consultation

Norma was encouraged to discuss contraception for the future: it was agreed that she should be fitted with an IUCD in the near future, and that, in the meantime, her husband should use a sheath. Advantage was also taken at this contact to check that Duncan had a date in the near future to attend the well-baby clinic for screening and immunizations.

(c) Follow-up arrangements

Norma was asked to make an appointment to be seen again in about 5 weeks, irrespective of other arrangements that might or might not be made about fitting a coil.

Further reading

GUILLEBAUD, J. (1983). Postcoital contraception: patients' questions answered. *Modern Medicine*, **28**, 69–70

Presentation 17: Sandy, aged 18 months; a rash in a child who is not ill, seen on a home visit

(a) Measles?

This diagnosis is usually more readily formulated by parents than by doctors – hence a verbal story that a child has already had measles often needs to be accepted by the doctor with mental reservations. In Sandy's case, the lack of a significant prodromal catarrhal phase and an alert-looking child who is not apparently off his food make this diagnosis less likely. A quick check to ensure that Koplik's spots are not present will further assist in the exclusion. It is just possible that Sandy may have developed partial immunity to measles from previous vaccination, and a check of his records (if any) regarding immunization status may help.

(b) Possible alternative diagnoses

Rubella is a possibility and it would be worth seeking collateral clinical evidence from the distribution and nature of the rash, together with a purposeful search for occipital lymphadenopathy. A number of different viruses, mainly of the enteropathic group, may give rise to the rather nondescript clinical picture Sandy exhibits. One feature of note, however, is the distribution of the rash on the face. Even as an isolated phenomenon, this clinical feature suggests the possibility of erythema infectiosum, 'slapped-cheek' disease or so-called 'fifth disease'. Faced with a crop of similarly afflicted children in his practice, the general practitioner is on firmer ground in making such a diagnosis. Recent work (Anderson *et al.*, 1983) suggests that human parvovirus infection is a probable aetiological agent. Whatever the diagnosis, the condition is one that is likely to be self-limiting within a few days.

(c) Follow-up arrangements

New entrants to general practice usually have to learn the need for the doctor to 'draw the line' under an episode of illness, and signal to the patient or, as in Sandy's case, the parents in a positive way that an episode of illness may be considered 'closed'. Failure to do this firmly may lead to unnecessary prolongation of 'illness' – long after the disease has vanished. In Sandy's case it might be enough to say, 'I expect he'll be as right as rain in a couple of days – why not give me a ring to tell me, or sooner if you think it appropriate?'.

(d) Other action

Each contact with a patient may be used in ways to extend the care the doctor can give (N. Stott, 1983). In Sandy's instance, the doctor might compare his behaviour and development (sitting up and alert) with what he would expect of a normal child of Sandy's age. This informal unobtrusive 'developmental scanning' may be just as effective as massive strategic screening endeavour – and so very much cheaper.

Further reading

ANDERSON, M.J., JONES, S.E. *et al.* (1983). Human parvovirus, the cause of erythema infectiosum (fifth disease)? *Lancet*, **i**, 1378

CAMPION, P.D. and KNOX, J.D.E. (1984). A difficult case: disengagement from medical care. *British Medical Journal*, **288**, 293–294

MORRELL, D. (1982). The patient complaining of a rash. In *Practice – a Handbook of Primary Medical Care*. Eds. J. Cormack, M. Marinker and D. Morrell. London: Kluwer Medical. Ch.3.27

STOTT, N.C.H. (1983). *Primary Health Care*. Berlin: Springer Verlag

Presentation 18: Ethel Smith, in her fifties, with a blood blister

(a) Emotionally charged words

(i) Words like 'spine' instead of 'back' or 'backbone', or 'agony' in place of 'pain', 'collapse' for 'faint', are additional examples. Sometimes the lay use of a technical term (especially the incorrect use) has the same effect, as in the expression 'I've got a gastric stomach'. Doctors need to beware of unwittingly provoking defensive reactions in patients by inappropriate use of emotionally charged words when obtaining a history (Froelich and Bishop, 1972).

(ii) The use of such terms may be the expression of anxiety – fear of the unknown. Sometimes the patient may use such terms to impress the doctor with his knowledge. Occasionally such terms are used to manipulate the doctor into according a higher priority to the request than he might otherwise do. The newcomer to general practice needs to acquire a 'nose' for this aspect of work if he is to be an efficient as well as an effective doctor.

(b) Extent of physical examination

Extending the notion of efficiency, all clinicians and especially those in general practice acquire a 'streamlining' in their clinical method. Where physical examination is concerned, this matching of its nature and extent to the situation presents peculiar problems to the newcomer to the 'minor medicine' of general practice; 'streamlining' may be confused with 'cutting corners'. In Miss Smith's case, for example, a rectal examination is unlikely to provide significant positive or useful negative information. History and local examination of the mouth are all that are required to provide a 'provisional formula for action'.

(c) Management of traumatic oral submucosal haematoma

The sooner the blood blister is evacuated, the smaller will be the area denuded of mucosa. The blister is punctured by a needle and the blood gently expressed. In Miss Smith's case, however, a relatively large area is already involved and she is likely to develop a painful shallow ulcer which will probably heal within a few days.

As is often the case with 'minor medicine' (*see p.53*), it is the meaning the condition may have for the patient which is the critical factor, rather than the physical discomfort from the condition itself. Miss Smith needs to be given the opportunity, therefore, to communicate the anxiety she had already expressed in her use of the word 'haemorrhage'.

Some doctors may not have encountered the well-defined, but not so well-known traumatic oral blood blister before, and might understandably feel insecure in making a diagnosis. Communicating doubts about possible coagulation disorders or other blood dyscrasias is unlikely to allay Miss Smith's fears.

Firm reassurance may be combined with a suggestion that she lets you know if she's still uneasy tomorrow. She could be instructed to manage any future such blisters herself by piercing them as soon as they appear. She will thereby lessen the chance of postblister ulcer.

Some patients are prone to repeated episodes for reasons not fully understood.

Further reading

FROELICH, R.E. and BISHOP, F.M. (1972) *Medical Interviewing,* 2nd edn. St Louis: The CV Mosby Company

Presentation 19: Mr McLeod, aged 81 years; a syncopal attack

(a) Assessing urgency

This is an important element in the day-to-day work of the receptionist (*see p.104*) who, in the past, has had to acquire the necessary skills the hard way without proper training, but this situation is slowly being rectified in the training courses now becoming more widely available in Colleges of Commerce and elsewhere in the UK.

In terms of probabilities Mr McLeod is most likely to have suffered a 'drop attack'. Although alarming, such a syncopal episode is not usually associated with permanent neurological deficit but, as in Mr McLeod's case, physical trauma may be associated with the fall.

That your receptionist has passed on the message immediately, however, introduces the opportunity for you to act on the high priority implicit in her interruption of your consulting – and you cannot be sure at this stage whether there may be more sinister pathology behind Mr McLeod's 'collapse'. Your receptionist's assessment will include the degree of pressure put on her by the relatives, together with her personal knowledge (which may be remarkably extensive and always of practical value) of the 'illness behaviour' of members of the practice and those associated with your patients, even if they are not on your NHS list.

(b) Selective awareness of clinical phenomena

While it may be possible for a clinician working in a narrow specialty to keep all elements of his clinical expertise at an equally high state of alertness all the time, most doctors, especially general practitioners, do not. Awareness is heightened selectively by a number of factors, important among which is the clinical setting.

In Mr McLeod's situation, such awareness would include attention to the possibilities of extensor plantar responses, extreme tachycardia, other abnormalities of cardiac rate and/or rhythm, bleeding from the ear, or other evidence of fractured skull.

(c) Adjusting levels of dependence

Mr McLeod will most likely wish to maintain his independence at home. His neighbour sounds as if she may not be so willing to share to the same extent Mr McLeod's desire. It is probable that further drop attacks are in the offing. Perhaps a relative might be available and willing to share the responsibility of keeping an eye on Mr McLeod, and a home help could be arranged on a once- or twice-weekly basis. Such steps might buy time to allow Mr McLeod to come to terms with the wrench associated with a move to sheltered housing, which might be an appropriate next line of support.

In areas fortunate enough to have a geriatric service which is 'prophylactically orientated' this might be a suitable opportunity to involve the local geriatrician and so minimize the disturbance often associated with later 'crisis intervention'.

Other things being equal, talk of a residential home for the elderly, or consideration for placement in a geriatric long-stay hospital would be inappropriate at this stage, unless it were initiated by Mr McLeod.

Further reading

HAMDY, R.C. (1984). Accidental falls. In *Geriatric Medicine*. London: Baillière Tindall. p.13
THOMPSON, M.K. (1980). Care of the elderly. *Update*, **21**, 571–584

Presentation 20: Bill Jones, aged 19 years; sore throat and malaise, seen at his house on a Saturday afternoon

(a) Factors governing the management of Bill's problem

Management depends on diagnosis which, especially for the general practitioner, requires a blending of physical, psychological and social considerations.

(i) *Physical factors.* On the evidence so far presented, Bill has at the least a good-going tonsillitis of the kind possibly associated with β-haemolytic streptococcal infection. However, the clinical finding of palatial petechiae strongly suggests glandular fever, a diagnosis rendered even more likely by his age. Bill was found to have splenomegaly in addition, so the diagnosis of infectious mononucleosis now becomes probable. Bill is thus likely to be in for a miserable week or two, and to require nursing care.

(ii) *Psychological factors.* It sounds as though Bill has been forced to admit defeat. Glandular fever does not suddenly develop at 3 p.m. on a Saturday afternoon, and it is probable that he has been attempting to struggle on for a few days against increasing disability. It also sounds as though he has problems of relationships at work – and there is the background of possible emotional reaction (akin to bereavement) at the break-up of his parents' marriage.

(iii) *Social factors.* Bill is clearly unfit for work on medical grounds. It is possible to leave him to attempt to cope on his own overnight until his father returns, though it is doubtful that his dad will be able to contribute much, wearied by his journey and with a home-coming on a Sunday.

It sounds as though admission to the local infectious diseases hospital might be an appropriate solution, to be discussed with Bill. You might want to consider how you might help him in contacting a responsible relative/neighbour to look after the house in the meantime: and a note for his employer, though *not* required for statutory sickness benefit, might just ease what sounds to be a difficult work situation.

(b) Responding to telephone calls

NHS regulations do not require the doctor to rent a telephone, though it would be a most odd kind of general practitioner who did not have one!

It is up to the doctor to decide, on the evidence provided by the caller, whether to visit or not. In non-emergency situations, the Health Departments encourage patients to put in requests for house calls in the early forenoon, preferably before 10 a.m. in the interests of the smooth running of the service.

In Bill's case, the doctor would have been within his rights to have refused to respond to his request – but the case illustrates the maxim 'when in doubt – visit'. Other considerations, in addition to need, demand and urgency, include geographical location and, perhaps more important, driving time, as well as the doctor's other commitments (as here).

Further reading

DRURY, M. (1981). *The Medical Secretary's and Receptionist's Handbook,* 4th edn. London: Baillière Tindall

Presentation 21: Grace P, an octogenarian, seen on a routine visit to a residential home for the elderly

(a) Long-term medication

Residents in old folk's homes are relieved of a number of responsibilities. This usually includes responsibility for drug therapy. In Mrs P's case, matron usually sends the doctor a request which is processed through the practice repeat prescription system. This consists of a chart kept in the patient's medical record listing the reasons for prescribing, the formulation, nature, strength, dose and amount of medication, together with dates of issue. The patient (or, in this case, matron) holds a patient repeat prescription card carrying similar data. On receipt of the request, the receptionist retrieves the case notes and writes out the medication on the prescription pad. The doctor checks the prescription against the chart and, if indicated, against the notes, ensuring that the patient has been seen by the doctor within a suitable period.

(b) Compliance

Staff of residential homes for the elderly are often faced with major problems in dealing with drugs. Studies have shown that each resident has, on average, three different preparations each requiring thrice-daily dosage. This means that in a home catering for 40 residents, staff have to cope with over 250 dosages per day. Ensuring the right dose of the right drug is given to the right patient from the right doctor at the right time can thus be seen to require a considerable degree of organization – and there is no statutory requirement, at the time of writing, for staff to hold nursing qualifications.

Some residential homes have systems of daily predispensing drugs into individual containers in each of three trays labelled 'breakfast', 'lunch' and 'supper', and delegate to a named staff member the responsibility of delivering the medication at table. Such a system may be backed up by a Kardex ledger containing the details of each resident's medication. The collaboration of a single retail pharmacist does much to ensure the smooth running of this system and a very high degree of patient compliance.

(c) Management

Consideration needs to be given to:

(i) Immediate issues, of which there are at least two: the urinary problems and pain relief. The advent of incontinence is important from the patient's point of view as yet another burden she has to bear; it may also be a factor in longer-term management decisions, should it prove to be persistent. Possible aetiological factors include infection, and/or incontinence from her inability to get to the toilet in time.

In addition to a search for infection, it would be worthwhile reviewing her analgesic therapy and, possibly, the hypnotic – oversedation might be a factor.

(ii) Longer-term management: appropriateness of her placement. It sounds as if Mrs P's problems have unobtrusively converted her into a patient with a high degree of nursing dependency. At the moment the staff do not appear to be making an issue of this aspect of her care, and Mrs P is unlikely to relish the prospect of a transfer to a long-stay geriatric hospital. Nevertheless, it would be appropriate to involve the local consultant in geriatric medicine in a review of Mrs P's condition.

Further reading

KNOX, J.D.E. and MELVIN, M. (1980). Prescribed medicines in a residential home for the elderly. *Nursing Times*, **76**, 1934–1936
NOYCE, P.R. (1982). Patient compliance. *Update*, **25**, 391–397

Presentation 22: Inappropriate housing for Miss Green, an octogenarian seen on a routine house visit

(a) Pathogenesis of locomotor impairment

On the limited information given, you would be justified in considering osteoarthrosis of the left hip as the likely disease process, associated with degeneration of articular cartilage, exposure of the underlying bone, which becomes denser, and localized overgrowth of bone round the periphery of the joint. At the age of 80 years, Miss Green may also be suffering from Paget's disease of bone and there is a strong likelihood of senile osteoporosis as well.

(b) Problem definition

Miss Green faces a number of problems including social and physical isolation contingent on her decreased mobility. The onset of senile dementia must raise doubts about her compliance with drug therapy, and with the advent of winter this elderly patient on thyroid replacement therapy is at special risk from hypothermia. It is an unfortunate fact that such an elderly person might also be at risk of being 'mugged'.

(c) Follow-up

It is likely that Miss Green's general practitioner will long ago have mobilized resources to maintain her independence in her own house for as long as possible. So, with a home help probably twice a week, a visit from the Nursing Sister (or one of her team) for a weekly bath, and neighbours or family encouraged to keep in touch, there is no pressing need for a frequent medical assessment. This is the sort of situation where, under normal circumstances, the doctor might look in, say, once a month or every 6 weeks. Unfortunately, when the pressure of work rises in general practice with, say, an epidemic of influenza or in the absence of a partner on holiday, visits to people like Miss Green are allotted a lower priority. Some doctors feel a sense of guilt about this: might such feelings be a factor in the doctor initiating the question of admission to long-term residential care for the elderly?

Further reading

GRAY, J.A.M. (1978). Housing, health and illness. *British Medical Journal*, **2,** 100–101

Presentation 23: Walter W, aged 48 years; a syncopal episode at home

(a) Physical diagnosis

(i) Such a fast apical rate strongly suggests the presence of paroxysmal tachycardia – and with a history of hypertension, ventricular tachycardia is a probability, as is shown in his electrocardiograph.

(ii) The absence of chest pain does not preclude a myocardial infarction which should be presumed to be the likely aetiological factor until proved otherwise. Such a rapid heart rate may well obscure characteristic ECG changes. Diagnosis of acute myocardial infarction can be difficult in general practice (van der Does, Lubsen and Pool, 1980).

(b) Immediate management

Among important considerations in Walter's care are the following physical, psychological and social factors:

(i) a rapid heart rate, calling for appropriate early specific therapy – possibly cardioversion

(ii) the likelihood of underlying infarction which, by now, is probably some 12 hours old

(iii) the need for higher dependency nursing care

(iv) the absence, at work, of his wife

(v) his wife's apparent unconcern, probably due to her failure to appreciate the potential gravity of the situation

(vi) the fact that both Walter and his wife have direct access to a telephone.

(c) Practice management issues

(i) The making of a tracing does not attract a fee for the NHS general practitioner.

(ii) As an independent contractor, the NHS general practitioner provides from his own funds such equipment as he may need, including an electrocardiograph.

Further reading

VAN DER DOES, E., LUBSEN, J. and POOL, J. (1980). Acute myocardial infarction: an easy diagnosis in general practice? *Journal of the Royal College of General Practitioners*, **30**, 405–409

Presentation 24: Mr Harold Green, an octogenarian on maintenance B$_{12}$ therapy, seen at home

(a) Prescription writing

The dispensing pharmacist requires data about the *recipient* of the prescription, the *medicine* and the *prescriber*, together with the date on which the prescription was written.

In Mr Green's case this would include his name and address: the doctor is not required to give the patient's age (although the age is required on NHS prescriptions for children under 12 years of age – as a safety measure). If Mr Green is obtaining his medicine free under NHS regulations (which is probable) he will be required to indicate that he is over pensionable age, and to countersign and date his prescription.

NHS prescription forms carry the letters 'NP' (*nomen proprium*) as a coded instruction requiring the dispensing pharmacist to indicate precisely the nature of the medication – in this case not simply 'the injection' but 'injection hydroxocobalamin'. The doctor may delete the letters if for any reason he does not wish to disclose the ingredients of his prescription.

Data concerning medication usually include the formulation (e.g. tablets, capsules, etc.), the drug, its strength, total amount to be prescribed and dose with instructions to the patient. This latter element in prescription writing is usually preceded by the term 'sig'. NHS prescription forms carry a box in which the doctor may indicate, where applicable, the number of days of treatment, thereby saving himself some mental arithmetic in calculating the total dose dispensed. The doctor's data include his professional address, signature and NHS code number.

Additional rules relate to the writing of prescriptions for scheduled drugs.

So Mr Green's prescription might be as follows:

Mr Green

    Harold

The Elms

    Inchgowrie

NP   No of days

℞

    Injection hydroxocobalamin 1 mg/ml
        Ampoules 1 ml × 5   [no instructions to the
                                       patient in this instance]

                     J Smith

                     A 1234

                     The Health Centre
                     Aberton

                     3.1.85

(b) Administration of B_{12}

The doctor has several options. He may delegate injection to a nurse of the primary care team. Intramuscular or subcutaneous injections usually are considered to be included in orthodox nursing procedures: furthermore, Sister can monitor Mr Green's condition professionally and check on his supplies of hydroxocobalamin. The nurse need not be the 'District Nurse' – Mr Green looks fit enough to attend the surgery premises where the practice nurse (*see* Presentation 30) could give him his injection. Secondly, the doctor may educate Mr Green to inject himself, as is common practice in the case of insulin-dependent diabetics. In doing this, of course, the doctor may lose the benefit of Sister's periodic professional assessment, and will therefore need some system to ensure both Mr Green's continued compliance with therapy and the continued professional monitoring of his well-being. Thirdly, the doctor may choose to give the injections himself, though it could be argued that the doctor's time might be put to better use.

(c) Additional doctor activity

As indicated *above*, in addition to administration of the maintenance hydroxocobalamin, there is the separate issue of monitoring Mr Green's well-being. This should include a routine clinical check to ensure the absence of anaemia and gastric symptomatology. Fraser, Cathcart and Sievewright (1983) advocate a once-yearly estimation of the haemoglobin level. Some would also suggest that Mr Green's serum calcium level should be checked periodically, in view of his previous history of partial gastrectomy and the known possible complication of osteomalacia.

(d) Gifts

One of the characteristics of general practice is the personal element in the doctor–patient relationship which, though not exclusively the prerogative of the discipline, may more often be developed to a higher degree than in other specialties.

In common with other branches of medicine, general practice affords opportunities for patients to express their gratitude for services rendered. Such giving and receiving of gifts may afford both parties pleasure in a transaction having an emotional basis. Sometimes however such actions may have a deeper significance, being a means of manipulating the unwary doctor. Some doctors too appear to have, as part of their make-up, a need to be met by the receiving of gifts – such doctors may actually boast about the number of bottles of whisky received at Christmas.

There may be other ways, more conducive to the patient's well-being, of satisfying this urge. One patient, for example, was encouraged to make an annual donation to the charity of his own choice!

Further reading

FRASER, R.C., CATHCART, M. and SIEVEWRIGHT, H. (1983). Audit of the use of vitamin B_{12} in general practice. *British Medical Journal,* **287,** 729–731
MARSHALL, S. G. and EKERSLEY, A. P. R. (1980). *A Primer of Primary Care.* London: Lloyd Luke

Presentation 25: Mrs Ambleside, aged 65 years, convalescent from myocardial infarction; seen to be deteriorating in adverse home circumstances

(a) Integrating physical, psychological and social factors

Physical factors in Mrs Ambleside's situation include possible effects of congestive failure, with decreased cerebral blood flow. She may be slowing up mentally (some patients undergo a personality change following a myocardial infarct), and poor compliance with her drug regimen is a possible result. Other psychological factors may be her unwillingness to volunteer possible urinary incontinence/infection unless specially afforded an opportunity to do so. Social factors include housing which, with its outside lavatory, does nothing to ameliorate Mrs Ambleside's problems. Additional factors include the increasing social isolation resulting from the alienation of the neighbour.

(b) Potential roles of the health visitor

The health visitor could carry out a more comprehensive assessment of the situation, ascertaining the view of the neighbour (who may not be your patient). In addition she could assist in management decisions for the longer term, while taking practical steps to ameliorate the immediate situation. Such steps could include increasing Mrs Ambleside's support by enlisting the help of any relatives and by mobilizing home help services and, possibly, meals on wheels. The health visitor could also assist in ascertaining the extent of Mrs Ambleside's compliance with drug therapy. She might obtain a urine sample for bacteriological examination. By her visits she could decrease Mrs Ambleside's social isolation and provide psychological support.

In planning for longer-term management, she might ascertain Mrs Ambleside's wishes regarding a possible move to sheltered housing; if such a move is agreed as desirable, she might provide the appropriate authorities with the necessary information, and initiate the move.

She could share follow-up visiting with the general practitioner in a co-ordinated manner, spacing out the contacts, possibly on an alternating basis.

Further reading

STANTON, A. (1979). A first experience of planning health visiting aims in a group practice. *Health Visitor,* **52,** 310–319

Presentation 26: Eliz Anderson, in her eighties, seen at home on her discharge from hospital after an acute respiratory infection

(a) Home from hospital

Most problems stem from the disruption of pre-existing arrangements for care in an on-going situation. This is one reason why it has been suggested that the term 'discharge' in relation to the elderly has become outmoded: 'transfer of care' is a more suitable phrase to describe the move. It is highly probable that Mrs Anderson's drug regimen, to which she had previously been accustomed, will have been amended by hospital doctors. Her former medication, if it has been continued, may have been substituted by the same generic drugs but in different formulations depending on the hospital's prescribing policy. New drugs may have been added to treat the temporary ailments. Sufficient supplies of drugs must be available for the short term. Arrangements for attendance at hospital follow-up clinic(s) may not be clear, especially the means of transport to be employed.

Sometimes patients in what is in effect a phase of convalescence require nursing assistance with personal hygiene: occasionally this is the start of a continuing nursing input to the on-going care of such elderly patients as Mrs Anderson.

Patients on arrival home from hospital sometimes experience an acute loss of confidence at the sudden deprivation of a constant readily available nursing presence.

During her admission, Mrs Anderson's home help will have been assigned to another needy person and arrangements will have to be made to restart the service. Mrs Anderson may be apprehensive at having lost the services of her familiar help and at having to 'break in' a stranger – fears that are often fully justified.

On a more practical level, milk and food supplies have to be restarted and if, as is the case with Mrs Anderson, the patient is too frail to do her own shopping, appropriate arrangements have to be made for her.

Some hospitals indicate their full awareness of all the factors mentioned *above* and attempt to involve the family doctor in a predischarge conference. Such occurrences, however, are the exception rather than the rule. Less rarely, the hospital makes some attempt before discharge to mobilize community resources so that they will become available to the patient soon after discharge. Sometimes such arrangements are left entirely in the hands of the general practitioner. Patients such as Mrs Anderson are occasionally given a hand-written note to pass to the general practitioner. Such communications detailing drugs, doses and diagnosis are usually followed up by a type-written conventional discharge letter. Patients (or their relatives) sometimes have a misplaced sense of the urgency concerning such provisonal communications, and this may have been a factor determining the decision to request a home visit to Mrs Anderson on a Saturday morning. Discharge home from hospital tends to occur more frequently at weekends, and Saturday mornings are not the easiest times for the general practitioner to start mobilizing support from the primary care team and the community.

(b) Doctor's aims in making this home visit

Since Mrs Anderson is well known to the practice, you would wish to make her feel welcome back home and to your care. She is likely to wish to give you a blow-by-blow account of her experiences in hospital. You will wish to know how she feels in herself, and will check her chest and possibly her abdomen. Each item of her medication should be checked against the hospital interim discharge letter and gone over with her to ensure she understands as far as possible the dose and the reason for each drug. If the hospital has given her a week's supply (as is common practice) you may wish to rationalize the containers to ensure that there is only one bottle for each medicine and to minimize possible confusion.

If appropriate, you may seek to contact your Nursing Sister in the community on the Saturday morning. Arrangements for home help will have to be left over to Monday; in the meantime you might contact the son to let him know you have visited and to enlist his support over the weekend. You will also indicate to Mrs Anderson that the practice will respond to any calls she may make over the weekend and that you will visit her again next week.

Further reading

STRANG, J.R., CAINE, N. and ACHESON, R.M. (1983). Team care of elderly patients in general practice. *British Medical Journal*, **286**, 851–854

Presentation 27: Florence Turner, aged 10 years, seen at home with a sore mouth and systemic upset

(a) Laboratory involvement in primary care

From the evidence – local lesions of the oral mucosa, systemic upset and paronychia – it is highly probable that Florence is suffering from primary herpetic gingivostomatitis and the concomitant finger lesion occasionally seen in this disease. An unusual feature is Florence's age, the disease being characteristically one of toddlers. Confirmation of the suspected diagnosis is probably an optional extra, because the diagnosis has been reasonably firmly established on clinical grounds, and drug therapy (including use of idoxuridine) is not likely to influence the natural history of the condition, which will run a self-limiting course over the next week or so. However, a swab may be taken from the mouth lesion, using a wooden shaft and broken into a bijou bottle containing virus transport medium. This, together with the appropriately completed form, must be transmitted as soon as possible to the virus laboratory (preferably within 6 hours). Unfortunately, because some otherwise apparently healthy 10 year olds normally harbour herpesvirus in their mouths, isolation of this virus does not *per se* prove the diagnosis. Further evidence in the form of a rising titre of antibodies needs to be forthcoming, so the swab should be accompanied by the first of a pair of blood specimens (10 ml whole blood in a plain tube). The second specimen should be obtained after an interval of a further 12–14 days.

A newer technique involves identification of circulating immune complexes from a single specimen of blood during the acute phase: it may be possible to identify from the complex the nature of the virus involved. However, the effort of entering this undertaking, which requires swabs, in-date transport media, invasive techniques and above all time, may be judged by the general practitioner to be insufficiently offset by information of practical value in management decisions regarding his patient.

Such considerations influence the use and non-use of laboratory help in the relatively minor medicine which forms such a large part of the general practitioner's clinical experience.

(b) Infectivity

From the above it will be clear that Mary is indeed at particular risk of picking up the infection. Spread is probably by direct contact with the virus excreted in the saliva, and the serial interval is about 10 days. Judging by the relatively low secondary attack rate of this condition, however, infectivity is not high, and it would be sufficient to ensure Mary does not use Florence's dishes or come into close contact until she is clinically well again.

(c) Prognosis

The condition is not amenable to therapy and the natural course of the clinical illness is about 10 days. Thus Florence will probably be able to take her exam, though she may still be feeling less than 100% fit.

Further reading

KNOX, J.D.E. (1968). 'Trench mouth' in children. *Journal of the Royal College of General Practitioners,* **12**, 23–30

Presentation 28: The late Mr Sidon – sudden unexpected death at home

(a) Urgent telephoned requests

Because of extreme anxiety to get the message across, the caller may ring off before giving the name and address. It is always worthwhile interrupting firmly and obtaining that vital information *first*.

To make speedy contact, among other things the doctor has to locate the address promptly. If he has previously visited the house this may present no problem, but if the address is unfamiliar, reference to a street map/directory *before he sets out* is obviously prudent. Information so obtained has to be applied with reference to the mad logic of urban address systems. Often (but not invariably) the locality will have some common theme to the naming of its streets, which are usually (but not invariably) numbered from the point nearest the civic centre, with even numbers on the left and odd numbers on the right.

On arrival, the doctor appraises the urgency by such features as an already open door and, at night, most of the house lights lit. There may be little knots of neighbours in the street or huddled in their doorways.

(b) Preparation for emergencies

For situations such as that involving the Sidons, most doctors keep an 'emergency bag'. The following is not a complete list of contents, but dealing with this situation might call for cardio-respiratory resuscitation – a Brook airway would be handy. Drugs and the means for their intravenous administration are necessary: depending on the diagnosis, these might include aminophylline, adrenaline, hydrocortisone, pethidine/morphia, anticonvulsants (e.g. diazepam) and glucose. It is worthwhile having an appropriate coin (currently 10p) to operate a public telephone (currently one in three households does not have a private telephone).

(c) Immediate moves – resuscitation?

Mr Sidon is 'obviously dead', probably signified by cessation of respiration, ashy cyanosis and fixed dilated pupils. To confirm this the doctor will wish to establish the absence of heart sounds and to examine the fundi for fragmentation of the blood columns in the vessels. Meantime he will be weighing up pros and cons of attempts at resuscitation. There is little point in attempting such moves if the pupils are dilated and fixed. Again, the doctor bears in mind the fact that Mr Sidon was a respiratory cripple; why attempt to drag him back to a life of crippledom, the next time to be terminated by the horrors of death from respiratory failure? On the other hand Mrs Sidon may have come to expect resuscitation as a routine practised by all doctors.

In addition to such considerations, the doctor will attempt to cope with Mrs Sidon's acute distress, remembering that she is not, technically, his patient.

(d) Cremation and sudden death

Before setting in train the arrangements for cremation, the doctor has to decide whether or not to issue a death certificate. Mr Sidon's is a sudden death though not, perhaps, an unexpected one. The cause is not obvious – possibilities include massive pulmonary infarction, acute myocardial infarction, and acute respiratory failure associated with postoperative respiratory infection. Postmortem examination alone will place the issue beyond doubt, but Mrs Sidon in her distraught state may not give 'informed consent'. If the doctor were to obtain a postmortem, cremation might still be possible, though funeral arrangements are likely to be delayed. The doctor has not seen Mr Sidon for some weeks prior to death. In England this means that the Coroner must be informed. In Scotland, however, this fact would not debar the doctor from issuing a death certificate if he felt reasonably certain about the likely cause.

In cases of doubt, however (and Mr Sidon comes into this category), external advice should be obtained. In Scotland, it is enough to discuss the situation with the local designated official, the Procurator Fiscal. In England, recourse must be made to the Coroner's office.

Postscript

Mr Sidon's case was even more complex because he had already bequeathed his body for anatomical dissection!

Further reading

CONSUMERS' ASSOCIATION (1967). *What to Do when Someone Dies*. London: Consumers' Association
GAULD, R.S. (1982). The role of the funeral director. *Update*, **24**, 85–88
KNIGHT, B. (1982). Sudden unexpected death. *Update*, **25**, 1507–1514
THE OXFORD GP TRAINEE GROUP (1979). *A Guide to General Practice*. Oxford: Blackwell Scientific Publications

Presentation 29: Alex Abel, aged 60 years; a late house call for 'a burn from an electric blanket'

(a) Fitness for work

The evidence suggests that Alex has in fact developed herpes zoster, probably affecting dermatomes left T6–7. In arriving at a decision as to his fitness, the doctor considers the following:

(i) At this stage Alex is likely to feel minor malaise combined with a burning discomfort at the site of his eruption. The disease usually runs a relatively benign course with vesicles crusting over within a week to 10 days. Postherpetic neuralgia is a possible complication afflicting about one in five patients.
(ii) His disease is not highly infectious.
(iii) His job as clerical officer is not likely to be physically demanding.
(iv) The missing evidence is how Alex and his wife see 'shingles' – some people tend to regard it as a major disaster, others shrug it off.
(v) There are only 3 working days left of this working week.

(b) Documentation

(i) As in all contacts with patients, the doctor should record clinical details in the medical record. Most general practitioners do not take the patient's record with them on an out-of-hours call such as this. The doctor may memorize the details and enter them next morning: some carry a small tape recorder and record the salient features at the time, for later transcription. Some practices, operating a rota system for out-of-hours cover, have developed a simple record card on which the details are entered and sent to the patient's personal doctor (if this is not yourself).
(ii) Medical certification for sickness benefit is not required unless more than 7 working days have been lost. Alex will require the appropriate 'self-certificate', supplies of which you would be wise to carry with you, although the onus is now on the patient to obtain the necessary form (from the local DHSS office among other places).
(iii) The whole episode appears to be a relatively minor one, and although agents such as amantadine–idoxuridine have their advocates, Alex probably needs nothing more than local

applications of talc and a regular dose of dispersable aspirin, so no prescription is strongly indicated on physical and pharmacological grounds. The doctor may need to take patient demand into account. After all, the Abel's have, themselves, seen Alex's 'illness' to be of such 'severity' as to justify an out-of-hours call on the doctor: to be fobbed off with a few aspirin as well as being 'put right' about a misdiagnosis may strain relationships.
(iv) If you wish to maintain the practice income, you are entitled to claim for a night visit fee. The appropriate form must be filled in, signed by the doctor (or authorized deputy) – but not now by the patient – and sent to the Primary Care Administrator (of the Family Practice Committee).
(v) Shingles, fortunately, is not a notifiable disease so you are spared that piece of documentation! Little useful purpose will be served by involvement of the laboratory at this time of night (if at all); so filling in laboratory forms and labelling specimen containers are not indicated.

Further reading

THE OXFORD GP TRAINEE GROUP (1979). *A Guide to General Practice.* Oxford: Blackwell Scientific Publications

Presentation 30: Sister Black, in the treatment room, at work on Mr Whyte's foot

(a) Foot conditions treated solely by a nurse

A wide range of conditions is theoretically possible but, in the case of an elderly gentleman, the list of the most likely conditions which Sister might deal with on her own includes routine care of the foot in diabetes mellitus, atheroma affecting large leg vessels, onychogryphosis, minor injury, and acute bursitis (bunion).

(b) Terms and conditions of nursing service

(i) Sister Black might be employed by the practice ('practice nurse') which pays her salary and reclaims 70% of it from the Primary Care or Family Practitioner administration under the NHS 'reimbursement of ancillary staff scheme'. Alternatively, Sister Black might be an employee of the Health Authority, who have granted her services as a 'practice-attached nurse'. This means that she ceases to owe her professional allegiance to a district, and instead provides nursing care for patients in the practice to which she is attached. Sometimes the literature conveys the impression that a Sister is attached to the doctor, and takes over his medical work. This is not so – her work is with the patients in the practice and comprises *nursing* duties. What constitutes nursing duties in the community gives rise to debate, because distinctions between medical and nursing needs of patients in general practice are sometimes much less clearly defined than in hospital.

(ii) From the *above*, questions of professional responsibility can be seen to be complex. The 'practice nurse', being an employee of the practice, could be considered accountable to the senior partner, acting under his direction, even though she may be seeing patients directly and without reference to or from NHS principals in the practice. The practice-attached nurse is in a rather different position, and may be held in a position of greater accountability. If she is acting in accordance with practice policy, she may also share professional accountability with doctors in the practice. She is also accountable to her superior nursing officer (District Nursing Officer).

(c) Pros and cons of different nursing managements

Doctors accustomed to working with 'their own' practice nurses are quick to point out the flexibility such an arrangement affords the practice in meeting patients' needs. Provided the employing doctor is satisfied that the nurse has been suitably trained for the task – from taking an ECG tracing to supervising the 'emergency bag' – she can get on with whatever tasks are agreed between them as appropriate for her. Disadvantages of the arrangement include the restriction (usually) of her work to the confines of the treatment room in the practice premises, and a degree of professional isolation.

Attached nurses, comparing their lot with their previous role of 'District Nurse', usually highlight the increased information about the patients and their families now available to them. Communications among members of the primary care team are increased and with this can come an increase in job satisfaction.

Attached nurses have not always been encouraged to develop the nursing element commonly presented by ambulant patients seen in the surgery premises, so they tend to continue to devote most of their time to domiciliary nursing care.

The presence of the two systems of management has tended to polarize into two factions what some would regard as the unity of nursing.

Problems may arise because of a mutual lack of understanding between the nursing administration (responsible for deploying nurses in the community) and the general practitioners. There are difficulties in attempting to marry a hierarchical type of management with the more egalitarian approach of general practitioners.

Further reading

HOCKEY, L. (1984). Is the practice nurse a good idea? *Journal of the Royal College of General Practitioners*, **34**, 102–103
McGREGOR, S.W., HEASMAN, M.A. and KUENSSBERG, E.V. (1971). *The Evaluation of a Direct Nursing Attachment in a North Edinburgh Practice*. Scottish Health Service Studies, No 18. Edinburgh: SHHD
POWELL, R.A. (1984). The Practice Nurse – a review. *Journal of the Royal College of General Practitioners*, **34**, 100–101
PRIMARY HEALTH CARE TEAM (1981). *Report of Joint Working Group of the Standing Medical Advisory Committee and the Standing Nursing and Midwifery Committee*. London: DHSS
REEDY, B.L.E.C., PHILIPS, P.R. and NEWELL, D.J. (1976). Nurses and nursing in primary medical care in England. *British Medical Journal*, **2**, 1304–1306

Presentation 31: Sally the receptionist, handing over a repeat prescription

(a) Functions of the receptionist

While the duties of the receptionist may be summed up as making first contact between patients and doctor, ensuring the smooth running of the consulting sessions and dealing with the telephone and medical records, the job is really an arduous one. For a fuller, first-hand account see Alkin (1982).

(b) Long-term drug therapy and osteoporosis

Problems inherent in Miss Gray's situation relate to non-effects, side-effects, over-effects and habituation. All non-steroidal anti-inflammatory analgesics carry risks which increase with the age of the patient, and Miss Gray is now in her eighties. Side-effects include peptic ulceration, inhibition of blood cell production, and skin rashes.

Her oral calcium preparation is relatively harmless, though Miss Gray has never been convinced that it has made much difference to her pain. Pain control in osteoporosis is seldom complete and the imperfections of drug regimens may account for the large number of preparations which are currently in vogue (*Drug and Therapeutics Bulletin*, 1984).

Insomnia, a normal accompaniment of old age, is aggravated by the constant pain Miss Gray suffers, yet it, too, is imperfectly controlled, even by a relatively high dose of benzodiazepine. It is likely that by now Miss Gray has become habituated to her therapy, with increased tolerance. She does run a risk of being more unsteady than she might be without her hypnotic, and a frail osteoporotic octogenarian is at special risk of incurring major fractures. On the other hand withdrawal of benzodiazepines is usually associated with a sense of increased malaise and tension which, however short-lived, will be poorly tolerated. The psychological effects of disturbing the 'balance' in some patients on long-term psychotropic medication have been vividly described by Balint and his colleagues (1970).

For these reasons the doctor has issued a repeat prescription.

(c) Repeat prescribing

The further issue of a prescription for medication which has already been continuously prescribed for 3 months or more falls within the definition of repeat prescribing.

This phenomenon, which hardly figured in studies of general practice in the 1950s, is on the increase due in part to the increase of the elderly in the population. It is an emotive subject, because some doctors insist that a patient must be seen by the prescriber each time a prescription is issued, and this makes other doctors feel guilty when, as in Miss Gray's instance, they do not see her. There is an element of confused thinking in relation to repeat prescribing, because there are two separate, though related, elements to it. The first is to make readily available to the patient, with a minimum of trouble to him or her, supplies of long-term medication. The second is to provide some form of monitoring of the patient and the drug situation. Professional assessment of the stabilized (or even healthy) patient can safely be separated from the issue of prescriptions, provided it is not forgotten. A system is needed to serve these different purposes. Many general practitioners issue repeat prescription cards to their patients, detailing drugs, their doses, duration of supply and date supplied (*see p.86*). The patient includes such a card in the written request for further supplies. The same details are entered in a repeat prescription chart (usually held in the patient's medical record). From this information the doctor can draw conclusions about the patient's compliance and decide when a further face-to-face contact is indicated. The advent of microcomputers has facilitated this activity, because they can print out the actual prescription and in addition provide a printed analysis of all repeat prescribing at the touch of a button (Meldrum, 1982).

Further reading

ALKIN, D.E. (1982). The role of the medical receptionist. *Update*, **24**, 2421–2424

BALINT, M., HUNT, J. *et al.* (1970). *Treatment or Diagnosis: a Study of Repeat Prescriptions in General Practice.* London: Tavistock Publications

Drug and Therapeutics Bulletin (1984). Osteoporosis. *Drug and Therapeutics Bulletin*, **22**, 1–4

MELDRUM, D. (1982). Repeat prescription control. *Update*, **25**, 2167–2175

Presentation 32: Gwen and her two children, Paul (2) and Barry (1), seen at the practice well-baby clinic

(a) Items of information on patients joining the practice

Of many useful items, perhaps the most salient concern any existing disease states and therapy (to ensure continuity of care) and possible emerging health problems (to plan for their avoidance or resolution). In the given situation, a number of issues need to be explored. Because they are sensitive personal matters, the doctor may wish to use time to allow them to emerge and then only after he has established a working relationship with Gwen and her family. In Gwen's situation, issues include current housing arrangements, plans and prospects regarding employment, and what support she may need (such as child-minding) while she settles in. Additional matters relate to factors inherent in her one-parent family situation – bereavement, separation or divorce? – and her reactions to probable trauma from such life events. Has there been a reactive depression, possible suicidal gesture or child abuse? From the photograph, the children appear well cared for, and the doctor will take the opportunity to check on the immunization status of each. Both Barry and Paul should by now have completed their courses of inoculations against diphtheria, tetanus and polio, as well as pertussis. Immunization against measles should be offered, if appropriate. In addition, the development of each child should be considered, even if only informally, at this stage, under the broad headings of posture and gait, fine movements, special senses, speech and social development. Because the practice runs its own 'well-baby clinic', the opportunity was taken at this first contact to introduce Gwen to Mrs Adams, the attached health visitor, to ensure more appropriate arrangements for periodic developmental assessment. Some practices request each adult joining the practice to complete a questionnaire covering items such as those mentioned above. Experience shows that information promptly gained in this way usually matches that eventually gleaned from the medical records when they become available and may give additional information not on record.

(b) Transmission of medical records

Under the NHS the organization responsible for administering family practitioner services undertakes to recall the medical records held by the practice with which the patient had registered previously and to transmit them to the 'new' doctor. A number of different steps are involved in this process, at each of which a time interval will elapse. When summated, these intervals may amount to months or even a year or more. If the doctor feels the need for immediate availability of information, the quickest way to obtain it is to telephone the patient's erstwhile general practitioner. The Family Practice Administrator of the area in which the patient has newly registered may, if requested, make special arrangements to expedite the transmission of medical records.

Further reading

DRURY, M. (1981). *The Medical Secretary's and Receptionist's Handbook,* 4th edn. London: Baillière Tindall

Presentation 33: a letter of complaint from RS, in the morning mail

(a) Assessing the situation

(i) The letter clearly conveys the writer's dissatisfaction with both your receptionist's behaviour and the quality of care provided by your practice. The writer is an intelligent, probably professional, man with some knowledge of medicine, and he is unlikely to let the matter rest.

(ii) Before taking action you would wish to obtain as full factual information as possible. This requires you to interview your receptionist. Staff loyalties are involved, as well as your personal responsibility (most, though not all, receptionists are employees of the partnership, not of the Health Authorities), and tact will be needed: you might wish to indicate that you know there is another side to the allegation. Your partner appears to have been involved, and you will wish to establish what, if anything, he can remember of the incident.

You will wish to know the medical background – the probability is that it is no more than undue panic about a breath-holding attack in the child of a psychologically disturbed family, but it could be more serious. You would wish to check the medical notes for any relevant entries relating to this episode and also to previous contacts (since these might assist in rebutting any charges of negligence). You might want to check the hospital side of the episode – was the child admitted, when, in what condition, and by whom? How is the child now? A brief telephone conversation with the consultant concerned may be indicated.

(b) Responding to the situation

The medicolegal undertones of this letter are so strong that whatever else you do you should send the original, keeping a copy, immediately to your Medical Defence Society. The letter should be accompanied by a factual *resumé* based on the moves you have made in (*a*) *above*.

You may be tempted to avoid face-to-face contact with the writer, and shelter behind some written response. This course is likely to aggravate a potentially difficult situation. A telephone call to him to arrange an informal face-to-face contact, preferably alone, might be in order; or you might wish to drop in on him 'out of hours' when he is likely to be at home. It would be important for you to keep a record of such an interview, but notes should not be made while you are interviewing him. It may be that this will be enough to cool the situation. Only after the heat has been taken out of the situation should the question of removal from the practice list be considered. This may best be done by a suggestion from you that, as it appears the practice has not met his expectations, perhaps he would wish to find another doctor. If, at a later date, the partners feel the need to protect the receptionist (assuming that this is a fair decision), then NHS regulations afford the right to request the appropriate NHS authorities to remove the family from your list.

Whatever the outcome, you would be wise to keep your Medical Defence Society informed.

Further reading

CALNAN, J. (1983). *Talking with Patients*. London: William Heinemann Medical Books
CONSUMERS' ASSOCIATION (1983). *A Patient's Guide to the National Health Service*. London: Consumers' Association and Hodder & Stoughton

Presentation 34: Elizabeth L's letter, received in the morning's mail, with an importunate request

(a) Medical report on Mrs L for life assurance

Mrs L is requesting the doctor to suppress information which she feels may operate to her disadvantage. The wording of her letter suggests that she realizes the unethical nature of her request; it is of interest to note the techniques she uses to gain her ends – exploitation of the personal relationship, persuasion, and intellectual justification. The use of the doctor's Christian name and the letter's personal tone are reinforced by the phrase 'would you be a pet . . .' together with hearsay evidence of the last hospital encounter.

The options open to the doctor when approached by Emblem Life Assurance are to give a factual account of Mrs L's medical condition including her enteropathy, or to decline to furnish any report. Ethical, and probably legal, considerations preclude 'compliance' with Mrs L's request.

The fact that she has requested suppression of part of her medical history does not imply the suggestion that you do not have her permission to disclose the facts. The life assurance company would be unlikely to approach you if it did not have that permission.

If you provide the usual report, you would be wise to ensure that you clearly mark the envelope 'To the medical officer' and endorse it 'Confidential'. Not all life assurance offices are as scrupulous in this observance, which should be universal practice irrespective of the nature of the report.

If you decline to furnish a report, you are likely to make life unnecessarily difficult for Mrs L.

(b) Mrs L's 'provisions'

Mrs L is likely to require supplies of gluten-free flour and foods. Normally, the NHS general practitioner may not supply, on NHS prescriptions, substances classified as foods. Gluten enteropathy is an exception, though the regulations concerning 'borderline substances' are not entirely straightforward. Thus, it is justifiable to prescribe gluten-free loaves, flour and crackers (unspecified). The designation of particular kinds of biscuits, however, is likely to result in the cost of such a prescription being referred back to the *doctor* to pay. The mechanism by which this is done is complex and involves the scrutiny to which all NHS prescriptions are subjected in the 'Pricing Bureau'.

Further reading

BRITISH MEDICAL ASSOCIATION (1984). *BMA Handbook on Medical Ethics*. London: British Medical Association
HAVARD, J.D.J. (1984). Protecting confidentiality. *British Medical Journal*, **288**, 1102–1103

Presentation 35: Letter from Mary Seton

(a) Selecting a general practitioner and joining the NHS list of patients

Remarkably little factual information appears to exist on the factors involved in the selection process. Common sense suggests that important considerations include being born into a family already registered, propinquity, recommendations of neighbours and friends, other personal advice (e.g. the views of the family doctor whose list the patient is leaving) and, probably most importantly, opportunistic need – an epidemic of illness in the practice will usually yield a crop of previously 'unregistered' patients. The general practitioner has a right to accept or refuse applications to join his list. In larger health centres, housing several different practices, a system usually operates whereby all casual enquiries concerning registering are channelled selectively to successive practices by rotation, over periods of a week or a month.

Registration of a patient depends on the receipt by the appropriate primary care (or family practitioner) administration of a form signed by both patient and doctor. This is one of the few instances in medical practice where the professional relationship is reinforced by a written contract between patient and doctor. The freedom of choice of doctor is an important element in British

NHS general practice and contributes to the special relationship characteristic of family doctoring. The choice is, of course, also governed by a number of other considerations such as the number of doctors available in a given locality and the list size.

(b) Mrs Seton's letter

The wording of the letter suggests that Mrs Seton may be significantly depressed: it also conveys an element of manipulation.

The question of why the letter was written when it was, raises possibilities such as: has Mrs Seton had a row with her doctor? or has the practice with which Mrs Seton is registered put her off their list of patients?

What are the possibilities if you agree to accept Mrs Seton back on your list? Might she have learned from the situation? Might your ready acceptance be in danger of being misinterpreted by the practice with which she is (so far as you know) registered? Might your partners, nursing and health visiting colleagues in your practice take a different view from you on the question of readmission to the list? If you refuse to take Mrs Seton back, might you contribute further to her depressed state: is suicide a possibility?

It was with such considerations in mind that the following reply was written:

Dear Mrs Seton,

Thank you for your letter letting me know how low you feel at present.

I have delayed replying to your request until I had had a chance to discuss the situation with my colleagues who work in the practice. After consideration we feel it would not be in either your best interests or ours for you to come on the list again.

With every good wish.

Yours sincerely,

YX

Presentation 36: Letter from an unknown
patient

(a) The writer

The writer's preoccupation with eating and body image ('ugly fat') indicate that the presentation concerns the group of conditions encompassed in the spectrum bulimia–anorexia nervosa. Sufferers from these states are usually girls in late adolescence. The strange spelling and syntax errors might be the result of poor or interrupted schooling, yet they are in contrast to the generally articulate nature of the letter. Though they are not in themselves of such gross degree to betoken dyslexia, they suggest someone writing under some distress and may even raise the possibility of psychotic disturbance which is an occasional feature of anorexia nervosa.

(b) Deciding on a response

(i)   The writer is not your patient in the sense of being registered with your practice, and it is highly probable that she is registered with a local general practitioner.
(ii) The condition from which she appears to suffer is one of extreme complexity (Kitson, 1984).
(iii) The writer indicates that very considerable therapeutic effort has already been exerted on her behalf. If, as is likely, she is in the middle of an on-going planned regimen, any uninformed intervention by yourself could unwittingly upset her management.
(iv) An appeal of this kind can be difficult to ignore, though your desire may be tempered by your own lack of expertise in this particular subject.

(c) One response

In the light of the above considerations, any response should be discrete and circumspect. Any commitment in writing should be an informed one, best made by taking her own general practitioner's views into account. To find out who the doctor is means the writer will have to be contacted, preferably by telephone. Since the letter-head carried no telephone number this information was obtained from Directory Enquiries.

The writer was contacted and turned out to be a well-spoken 21-year-old unmarried woman. After preliminary discussion, she readily agreed that her general practitioner should be contacted by telephone. The doctor confirmed suspicions that Miss C S had indeed had a very stormy time, having had repeated psychiatric in-patient therapy for her anorexia nervosa. She was in fact under continued care by both the family doctor and the psychiatric clinic.

Under these circumstances, the following written reply was sent to Miss C S and a copy sent to the general practitioner.

Miss C S
Bogle Farm
Abbeyton
Northington

Dear Miss S,

First of all, thank you for taking the trouble to write about your distressing complaint. I appreciate that you must have gone through a pretty difficult time and can understand that you would wish to explore new treatments that might appear to offer some relief. The operation you mention is sometimes carried out in very special circumstances. I have no first-hand experience but I know that there are a number of snags to it.

As we discussed on the telephone, I am sure that your next move should be to discuss the situation with your doctor, to whom I am sending a copy of this letter. I have already been in touch with him and I know that he has your interests very much at heart.

With all good wishes.
Yours sincerely,

Further reading

KITSON, N.I. (1984). Why are anorectics so difficult to treat? Update, **28**, 1311–1315

Part III

One-to-one teaching in the practice

Introduction to Part III

One-to-one teaching in medical practice is not new and the apprentice nature of training is depicted in such paintings as Goya's 'El medico'. It is only within the last two decades, however, that the nature, content and methods especially appropriate to training in general practice have been more clearly defined. The book *The Future General Practitioner – Learning and Teaching* (RCGP, 1972) remains an important landmark. Comparatively little has so far been written about the practicalities of teaching and learning on a one-to-one basis in a practice setting, so the following contributions are aimed at filling this gap. The first essay is concerned with fitting the trainee into the practice, while the second describes a tutor's handling of an undergraduate's attachment.

Experience, documented by Richardson (1970), Wright (1974) and others, shows that patients in general practice have accepted the teaching situation, provided it is handled with tact. The patients' wishes must be taken into account. Some teachers have found that sometimes these views go beyond a mere passive acceptance of a situation in which patients may be used for teaching: it is possible for the teacher to engage in a more active relationship, enhancing the potential teaching role of the patient inherent in most general practice consultations. Teaching of communication skills is particularly well suited to this development (Kent, Clarke and Dalrymple-Smith, 1981; Murdoch, 1982).

A trainee in the practice: the early days

Preliminary steps

Long before the trainee is actually fitted into the practice, a number of preparatory steps will have been taken by the practice to meet the local and national requirements for training. In obtaining approval of the General Practice Sub-committee of the Regional Postgraduate Education Committee, for example, the intending trainer will have demonstrated his own personal abilities both as a doctor and as a potential teacher. The practice will have been inspected: the adequacy of the premises to accommodate the trainee, attitudes of partners and staff towards vocational training, the medical records, practice library facilities and other adjuncts to the business of training will all have come under scrutiny. Most teaching practices will also have considered the possible effects on patients of having a trainee in post. A leaflet indicating that the practice is becoming involved in teaching and that a new doctor will be joining the team can be made available to patients at reception – or the information can be incorporated into a newsletter where this is appropriate. The practice 'grapevine' will, no doubt, be busy!

The intending trainee, too, will have taken a number of steps before actually joining the practice. Entry into training is broadly through two main channels: by appointment to a training scheme with its package of hospital appointments and training practice; or by direct application to an approved training practice as part of a 'self-constructed' plan. Since this article is primarily concerned with educational considerations once the trainee has actually arrived in the practice, the reader wishing further details of these preliminary steps is referred to such guide books as those by Fry (1982) or Hall (1983).

Forrester (1984) suggests that it is in the best interests of all concerned that a prospective trainee should spend half a day in the practice *before* arrangements are finalized: his assessment is based on a relatively informal approach which he and his partners have found to be worthwhile.

Early days

It is natural that, at first, the trainee should feel apprehensive, and the same may be true of the trainer, especially if he is a newcomer to teaching. One way of easing the situation is for both parties to set aside time to discuss such basic issues as where the trainee will work, his timetable, commitment to care of patients, including out-of-hours arrangements, and the provision of equipment he will need. Making the first of these discussion sessions a social occasion, say, by inviting the trainee to meet the trainer's family at a meal, can be a useful start. Such an introduction can also afford an opportunity for an additional unobtrusive 'assessment'; the family's observations of the trainee may sometimes provide the trainer with helpful guidance in devising the early stages of the training programme. An informal setting, too, can encourage the trainee to share problems and anxieties regarding such basic housekeeping issues as his living accommodation, telephone call arrangements, and so on. The trainee needs to know to whom he can turn at any time when he is on duty, and this support is especially important during the early days in the practice. The level of anxiety can be lessened by providing an outline of the sort of activities in which the trainee will be involved, and their timing. It is easy to slip too readily into a fixed timetable, the rigidity of which may later interfere with learning opportunities – so the provisional nature of the timetable should be stressed at the outset. The one exception to this is the trainee's half-day which ought to be a fixed and regular entity – even if this does not apply to the trainer!

In the first few days the main educational activity will be assessment – this is a two-way affair, however it is performed, whether consciously or unconsciously, formally or informally.

Pretraining assessment

Each trainee will bring to the situation educational needs (and strengths) which will vary widely between one doctor and another. Because virtually all UK medical schools now incorporate some contribution from general practice into the undergraduate curriculum, the nature and range of variation of the trainee's needs are changing, but most beginners still demonstrate, in their approach to patients, a hospital orientation, with hallmarks such as: preoccupation with disease; failure to appreciate the significance of social and psychological elements and their bearing on, especially, management; and difficulty in tolerating uncertainty, in the face of the need to be effective clinically.

The trainer needs to obtain some idea of these (and other) characteristics because they provide important teaching and learning opportunities round which the training curriculum may be devised. This kind of assessment needs to be supplemented by the identification of gaps in factual knowledge and clinical skills. The trainer new to teaching may be tempted to take too much for granted in this important part of training.

Some indication of the trainee's needs at the outset can be obtained by observing him in consultation, by paper exercises (such as those provided by *Part I* of this book) and by the use of checklists. Reed (1984) provides a convenient 'pocket examiner' which could be used for this purpose.

Sitting in on consultations

Some of the inquisitional nature of this form of assessment can be reduced by agreeing to exchange the observer role between trainer and trainee from time to time. This is an important part of training and should be used both at the start and, periodically, *throughout* the training period, involving consultation on the surgery premises and at home visits. Observations by both trainer and trainee of each other's behaviour (and of the patient) made on these occasions may then form the basis of short tutorials.

Some trainers make a point of sitting in on all the trainee's consultations until satisfied that the doctor has demonstrated abilities to cope with basic and common issues. This may take about a week, but there is no statutory period before a trainee 'goes solo'. By the same token, before involving the trainee in the more salient experiences of decision-making in out-of-hours work, trainers will usually arrange to accompany their trainees on the first two or three night calls. Often the practical problems of providing direct telephone links to the trainee's house deprives the learner of first-hand experience of this important part of patient management, and the trainer will need to consider how best to plug this gap if it should exist.

Self-recording and classifying contacts

A function of training is to create a greater awareness of the patient and his circumstances in relation to health problems. It should be possible for the trainee to demonstrate his progress along this path by recording details of consulting sessions and then attempting to classify the contacts along the lines given in *Part II* of this book (*p.53*). The hypothesis is that, as he progresses through training, a trainee's appreciation of the complexities will be expressed by a greater proportion of contacts in categories other than 'simple minor'. By the same token, his management actions should show a greater proportion of activities at levels III, IV and V (*see p.51*). The trainer may need to engineer the trainee's consulting so as to ensure an appropriate mix of the more complex 'minor medicine'.

Constructing a curriculum

Depending on the results of assessments obtained by the methods described and in other ways, modifications can be made to the basic pattern of consulting, time off, the day-release, half-days, etc. It is always worthwhile having the trainee spend a session acting as receptionist, filing clerk, or other member of the secretarial team. This is probably best arranged during the early phase in the practice and is one way in which the trainee, staff and patients can rapidly become acquainted with one another. Similar sessions should be arranged with other practice staff, such as health visitor and nursing Sister. Such sessions can help to orientate the trainee both professionally and geographically.

Introducing the trainee to the local retail pharmacist, the clergy and the undertaker usually has to be a more active process than is introduction to colleagues in hospital, and is equally important.

Project work

Before the trainee settles into a routine, consideration should be given by both trainer and trainee to the possibility of the trainee carrying out a study of some aspect of his work in general practice. An important factor determining the choice of topic should be the trainee's preference, and he may need a little time – say, the first few weeks – to become aware of the wide range of subjects open to him. He could be encouraged to pursue original ideas by allocating a set time weekly for such work. Help and advice in planning will be forthcoming from sources such as the local University Department of General Practice or from the Royal College of General Practitioners.

Back-up

Both trainer and trainee do not work in a vacuum – the training in the practice is, or should be, part of a wider educational endeavour. Regular contact should be maintained with the day-release course, with the trainers' workshop and with those having oversight of training arrangements – course organizer and Regional Adviser in General Practice.

Final-year student attachment in rural practice: a tutor's view, *by the late* *A.G. Reid* FRCGP MBE

It is helpful if the student can arrive at a time when he (she) can be interviewed at leisure before seeing patients. The practice can be described and plans outlined. An assessment can be made of the student's previous experience and attitudes, and likely knowledge gaps or special interests discussed.

It is well to warn the student – not too seriously – that he will inevitably be somewhat bewildered by the first day or two, with so many new contacts, and that he will regard the apparent negligence of his tutor with horror. This is assuming, as it is with us, that it is the student's first visit of this kind to a practice. Differences from hospital can be discussed and the tutor's knowledge of the previous history and background of the majority of the patients emphasized. What one can teach is largely determined by what crops up during the attachment.

The student will probably be surprised at the amount of serious organic disease that is being seen, and this should be stressed. The very long-term regular care required by many such patients, and that such patients with definite diseases are frequently comparatively easy to deal with so long as the home conditions are stable and good, can be demonstrated. Terminal care, perhaps ending in the Cottage Hospital, will be included in this.

One increasing difficulty will become obvious, however, and that is the complexity of therapy as ill patients live longer – not the treatment of hypertension, or of hypothyroidism, or of depression, but the juggling required to treat all three in one patient.

Many of these patients will be seen at home, and car journeys between calls can serve as tutorial sessions.

Emergency calls will bring to the student an awareness of the factors which may lead to a hospital admission, or to observation at home, and give an opportunity to discuss the pros and cons of home *versus* hospital in, for example, myocardial infarction.

The impact of an event like infarction in a wage-earner can be shown, and the tutor's respect for his patients as people and his 'empathy' with the family made evident. But the need for objectivity must also be stressed.

Ideally, an attempt should be made to extend consulting times to give an opportunity for a briefing and discussion on most patients. In the consulting room the student may be given a simple recording project, perhaps reflecting his particular interests. Students vary widely in their experience of even simple procedures, and may have to be instructed in the use of, for example, an auriscope. Nothing should be taken for granted. Practical procedures such as injections and venepunctures should be minutely supervised *after* demonstration, to ensure that the patients are not upset.

Receptionists should inform patients on arrival that a senior student is with the doctor and give an opportunity for the patient to object. This almost never happens and no difficulty is ever experienced on visits to the homes. It is wise to arrange a code phrase with the student, such as 'Will you check the sterilizer, please', if the student's presence is felt to be making things awkward. Again, this is rarely needed.

As time passes, students should be asked to examine the patient first and 'be the doctor', but correction and discussion should be discreet in front of the patient, and the student should not be made to appear incompetent. He should be made to understand that your silence means, 'We shall discuss this later'.

It is generally easy to leave the student with the patient, perhaps as you deal with a phone call. Animated conversation as you return suggests ability to communicate but it may, of course, be initiated by a helpful patient.

If transport can be arranged an eager student may usefully visit one or two families for an extended time.

Practice administration, records and repeat prescribing will all come up for discussion, especially with those heading for practice.

It can be pointed out that on many of the commonest subjects there is no real consensus of opinion, for example, treatment of sore throats, or hypertension, and there is room for differences of opinion; pragmatic activity in the light of the patient's individual situation is required.

After a day or two, emphasis will have been placed on the total physical, psychological and social assessment of the patient. Concepts such as the extended consultation and probability diagnosis can be demonstrated, and one hopes that by the end of the attachment the student will feel the system makes sense.

It is important to be enthusiastic about practice, and to avoid too many grumbles about conditions and patients. The tutor may find himself in a therapeutic situation with the student's own problems and, properly handled and reported, this can be valuable. This may be more likely if the student is invited to share the tutor's family circle in the evenings.

Bibliography

ALKIN, D.E. (1982). The role of the medical receptionist. *Update*, **24**, 2421–2424

ANDERSON, M.J., JONES, S.E. *et al.* (1983). Human parvovirus, the cause of erythema infectiosum (fifth disease)? *Lancet*, **i**, 1378

BALINT, M., HUNT, J. *et al.* (1970). *Treatment or Diagnosis: a Study of Repeat Prescriptions in General Practice.* London: Tavistock Publications

BALINT, E. and NORRELL, J.S. (Ed.) (1973). *Six Minutes for the Patient: Interactions in General Practice Consultation.* Mind and Medicine Monographs, No.23. London: Tavistock Publications

BENNISON, J. and MARINKER, M. (1982). Changes in facial appearance. In *Practice – a Handbook of Primary Medical Care*. Eds. J. Cormack, M. Marinker and D. Morrell. London: Kluwer Medical. Ch.3.14

BRITISH MEDICAL ASSOCIATION (1984). *BMA Handbook on Medical Ethics.* London: British Medical Association.

British National Formulary, No.8 (1984). London: British Medical Association and The Pharmaceutical Society of Great Britain. pp. 25–27

CALNAN, J. (1983). *Talking with Patients.* London: William Heinemann Medical Books

CAMPION, P.D. and KNOX, J.D.E. (1984). A difficult case: disengagement from medical care. *British Medical Journal*, **288**, 293–294

CONSUMERS' ASSOCIATION (1967). *What to Do when Someone Dies.* London: Consumers' Association

CONSUMERS' ASSOCIATION (1983). *A Patient's Guide to the National Health Service.* London: Consumers' Association and Hodder & Stoughton

COURTENAY, M.J.F., CURWEN, M.P. *et al.* (1974). Frequent attendance in a family practice. *Journal of the Royal College of General Practitioners*, **24**, 251–261

DHSS (1983). *Medical Evidence for Social Security and Statutory Sick Pay Purposes.* London: DHSS

Drug and Therapeutics Bulletin (1984). Osteoporosis. *Drugs and Therapeutics Bulletin*, **22**, 1–4

DRURY, M. (1981). *The Medical Secretary's and Receptionist's Handbook*, 4th edn. London: Baillière Tindall

126

ENELOW, A.J. and SWISHER, S.N. (1972). *Interviewing and Patient Care*. London: Oxford University Press. Ch.4

EUROPEAN CONFERENCE ON THE TEACHING OF GENERAL PRACTICE (1977). The work of the general practitioner – Leeuwenhorst Working Party Report. *Journal of the Royal College of General Practitioners*, **27**, 117

FORRESTER, A.G. (1984). Assessing a prospective trainee. *Journal of the Royal College of General Practitioners*, **34**, 407

FRASER, R.C., CATHCART, M. and SEIVEWRIGHT, H. (1983). Audit of the use of vitamin B_{12} in general practice. *British Medical Journal*, **287**, 729–731

FREELING, P. (1983). *A Workbook for Trainees in General Practice*. Bristol: Wright

FREELING, P. and HARRIS, C.M. (1984). *The Doctor Patient Relationship*, 3rd edn. London: Churchill Livingstone. p. 60

FROELICH, R.E. and BISHOP, F.M. (1972). *Medical Interviewing*, 2nd edn. St Louis: The C V Mosby Company

FRY, J. (1982). *Guide for Trainees in General Practice*. London: William Heinemann Medical Books

GAULD, R.S. (1982). The role of the funeral director. *Update*, **24**, 85–88

GRAY, D.J. Pereira (1979). The key to personal care. *Journal of the Royal College of General Practitioners*, **29**, 666–678

GRAY, J.A.M. (1978). Housing, health and illness. *British Medical Journal*, **2**, 100–101

GUILLEBAUD, J. (1983). Postcoital contraception: patients' questions answered. *Modern Medicine*, **28**, 69–70

HALL, M.S. (1983). *A GP Training Handbook*. London: Blackwell Scientific Publications

HAMDY, R.C. (1984). Accidental falls. In *Geriatric Medicine*. London: Baillière Tindall. p. 13

HANNAY, D.R., BARBER, J.H. and MURRAY, T.S. (1976). Attitudes towards the content of general practice teaching. *Medical Education*, **10**, 374–377

HAVARD, J.D.J. (1984). Protecting confidentiality. *British Medical Journal*, **288**, 1102–1103

HOCKEY, L. (1984). Is the practice nurse a good idea? *Journal of the Royal College of General Practitioners*, **34**, 102–103

JACKSON, C.R.S. (1975). *The Eye in General Practice*, 7th edn. London: Churchill Livingstone

KENT, G.G., CLARKE, P. and DALRYMPLE-SMITH, D. (1981). The patient is the expert: a technique for teaching interviewing skills. *Medical Education*, **15**, 38–42

KITSON, N.I. (1984). Why are anorectics so difficult to treat? *Update*, **28**, 1311–1315

KNIGHT, B. (1982). Sudden unexpected death. *Update*, **25**, 1507–1517

KNOX, J.D.E. (1968). 'Trench mouth' in children. *Journal of the Royal College of General Practitioners*, **12**, 23–30

KNOX, J.D.E. and CORMACK, J.J.C. (1982). Ankle and foot problems. In *Practice – a Handbook of Primary Medical Care*. Eds. J. Cormack, M. Marinker and D. Morrell. London: Kluwer Medical. Ch. 3.69

KNOX, J.D.E. and MELVIN, M. (1980). Prescribed medicines in a residential home for the elderly. *Nursing Times*, **76**, 1934–1936

Lancet (1984). Notes and News. Licensing restriction for prescription of dipipanone (Diconal). *Lancet*, **i**, 354

McGREGOR, S.W., HEASMAN, M.A. and KUENSSBERG, E.V. (1971). *The Evaluation of a Direct Nursing Attachment in a North Edinburgh Practice*. Scottish Health Service Studies, No 18. Edinburgh: SHHD

MADDISON, D.C. (1978). What's wrong with medical education. *Medical Education*, **12**, 97–102

MARSHALL, S.G. and EKERSLEY, A.P.R. (1980). *A Primer of Primary Care*. London: Lloyd Luke

MEDALIE, J.H. (1965). Levels of family practice and its implications for medical education. *Journal of the Royal College of General Practitioners*, **9**, (Suppl. 2), 20–30

MEDALIE, J.H. (1978). *Family Medicine – Principles and Applications*. Baltimore: Williams and Williams Co. pp.4–15

MELDRUM, D. (1982). Repeat prescription control. *Update*, **25**, 2167–2175

METCALFE, D. (1979). Education for co-operation in health and social work. *Royal College of General Practitioners, Occasional Papers*, No.14

MORRELL, D. (1982). The patient complaining of a rash. In *Practice – a Handbook of Primary Medical Care*. Eds. J. Cormack, M. Marinker and D. Morrell. London: Kluwer Medical. Ch. 3.27

MURDOCH, J.C. (1982). The patient as teacher. *Allgemeinmedizin International*, **11**, 26–27

NOYCE, P.R. (1982). Patient compliance. *Update*, **25**, 391–397

POND, D.A. and ESPIR, M. (1978). *Medical Aspects of Fitness to Drive*. Ed. A. Raffle. London: Medical Commission on Accident Prevention

POWELL, R.A. (1984). The Practice Nurse – a review. *Journal of the Royal College of General Practitioners*, **34**, 100–101

PRIMARY HEALTH CARE TEAM (1981). *Report of Joint Working Group of the Standing Medical Advisory Committee and the Standing Nursing and Midwifery Committee.* London: DHSS

REED, A. (1984). *Pocket Examiner in General Practice.* London: Pitman

REEDY, B.L.E.C., PHILIPS, P.R. and NEWELL, D.J. (1976). Nurses and nursing in primary medical care in England. *British Medical Journal,* **2,** 1304–1306

RICHARDSON, I.M. (1970). Patients and students in general practice. *Journal of the Royal College of General Practitioners,* **20,** 285–287

ROBINSON, E.H. and BARBER, J.H. (1977). Early diagnosis of pregnancy in general practice. *Journal of the Royal College of General Practitioners,* **27,** 335–338

ROYAL COLLEGE OF GENERAL PRACTITIONERS (1972). *The Future General Practitioner – Learning and Teaching.* London: British Medical Association

STANTON, A. (1979). A first experience of planning health visiting aims in a group practice. *Health Visitor,* **52,** 310–319

STOTT, N.C.H. (1983). *Primary Health Care.* Berlin: Springer-Verlag

STOTT, P. (1983). *Milestones – the Diary of a Trainee GP.* London: Pan Books. p. 129

STRANG, J.R., CAINE, N. and ACHESON, R.M. (1983). Team care of elderly patients in general practice. *British Medical Journal,* **286,** 851–854

THE OXFORD GP TRAINEE GROUP (1979). *A Guide to General Practice.* Oxford: Blackwell Scientific Publications

THOMPSON, M.K. (1980). Care of the elderly. *Update,* **21,** 517–584

TRING, F.C. (1977). Chilblains. *Nursing Times,* **73,** 1752–1753

VAN DER DOES, E., LUBSEN, J. and POOL, J. (1980). Acute myocardial infarction: an easy diagnosis in general practice? *Journal of the Royal College of General Practitioners,* **30,** 405–409

WALKER, E. and WILLIAMS, G. (1983). *ABC of healthy travel.* London: British Medical Association

WOOD, P.H.N. and BADLEY, E.M. (1981). *People with Arthritis Deserve Well-trained Doctors. The Report of a Workshop on the Medical Undergraduate Education in Rheumatology.* London: Arthritis and Rheumatism Council

WRIGHT, H.J. (1974). Patients' attitudes to medical students in general practice. *British Medical Journal,* **i,** 372–376

Index of topics